Men'sHealth

TNT DIET

Men'sHealth.

TNT DIET

TARGETED NUTRITION TACTICS

THE EXPLOSIVE NEW PLAN TO

BLAST FAT,
BUILD MUSCLE,

AND

GET HEALTHY

JEFF VOLEK, PhD, RD
AND ADAM CAMPBELL

RODALE

Men'sHealth

Library of Congress Cataloging-in-Publication Data

Volek, Jeff.
    Men's health TNT diet : the explosive new plan to blast fat, build muscle, and get healthy / Jeff Volek and Adam Campbell.
       p.   cm.
    Includes index.
    ISBN-13 978–1–59486–659–3   trade hardcover
    ISBN-10 1–59486–659–7   trade hardcover
    ISBN-13 978–1–59486–976–1   trade paperback
    ISBN-10 1–59486–976–6   trade paperback
    1. Weight loss.   2. Men—Health and hygiene.   3. Nutrition.   I. Campbell, Adam.   II. Title.
RM222.2.V56 2007
613.2'5081—dc22   2007023660

Distributed to the trade by Macmillan

2 4 6 8 10 9 7 5 3 1   hardcover
2 4 6 8 10 9 7 5 3 1   paperback

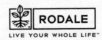

RODALE
LIVE YOUR WHOLE LIFE™

We inspire and enable people to improve their lives and the world around them
For more of our products visit **rodalestore.com** or call 800-848-4735

To the pursuit of eating well, looking good, and feeling great.

CONTENTS

ACKNOWLEDGMENTS

I could never properly thank all of the people who have contributed in some way to this book. But I'm particularly grateful to:

Steve Murphy and the Rodale family, to whom I extend my deepest appreciation for this great opportunity.

David Zinczenko: Thank you for your guidance, encouragement, and support.

The entire *Men's Health* book team, including Liz Perl, Nancy Hancock, Joyce Shirer, Claudia Allen, Zachary Schisgal, Courtney Conroy, Karen Neely, Kevin Smith, Chris Rhoads, Mitch Mandel, and Marc Sirinsky.

David Black, my agent.

Steve Perrine, Bill Stump, Peter Moore, Bill Phillips, Matt Marion, Bill Stieg, Lou Schuler, Tom McGrath, Ted Spiker, and Mark Bricklin: You have influenced and inspired me beyond measure.

Jeff O'Connell, Matt Bean, Scott Quill, Matt (Chef) Goulding, David Schipper, Erin Hobday, Denny Watkins, Alison Granell, Heather Loeb, Eric Rinehimer, Christine Maxfield, Jaclyn Colletti, Rob Gerth, Julie Lubinsky, Jeanne Emery, Charlene Lutz, Mary Rinfret, and Alice Mudge. I'm lucky to work with such a talented and hardworking group of people.

My friends and mentors: Alwyn Cosgrove, Bill Hartman, Michael Mejia, Robert dos Remedios, Craig Ballantyne, Chris Guinty, Jeff Simmons, Tim Stout, Craig Hope, Steve Hardin, and Pete "The Murge" Murges. Thank you for my continuing education—whether it be in training or in life.

Randy Milka, without whom this book would have never been written.

My coauthor, Jeff Volek: I value your friendship as much as your expertise. Thanks for all the biochemistry lessons and your tireless efforts to keep me motivated.

Don and Mary Nagle: The best in-laws a guy could have.

My bro, Craig, and my sister-in-law, Lori: Thank you for (truly) understanding me!

My sister, Beth Sweeny: You are always close to my heart.

My parents, Ray and Jane Campbell: The depth of my gratitude for your kindness, generosity, and unconditional love cannot be expressed here. Nevertheless, thank you for everything.

And, of course, my wife, Jessica, who endured months of "Sorry, honey, I have to work." You are my favorite.

—A.C.

This book is very much a synthesis of the collective scientific work I have conducted over the last decade and my own personal experiences with diet and exercise. First and foremost, the ideas espoused in this book are firmly grounded in metabolic and physiologic principles, and represent the collective expertise of many individuals whom I have interacted with during my scientific career. Although based heavily in science, thanks to my brilliant coauthor, Adam Campbell, the TNT Diet has now been transformed to its simplest core elements and translated so that even the most nonscientific individuals can understand and implement the plan. Thanks, Adam, without your persistence and heroic effort in putting these ideas to paper, this book would not be possible.

I have been fortunate to have many close friends and colleagues much smarter than me who have been instrumental in fueling my passion for discovery and molding my scientific perspective. William J. Kraemer, PhD, deserves special recognition. He introduced me to science serving as my major advisor through graduate school, and we currently work together as colleagues conducting research together at the University of Connecticut. I would not be the person I am today if I had not met Dr. Kraemer. I have the utmost admiration and respect for his determination and passion for mentoring students and research. It is truly an honor to be able to work so closely with such a preeminent scientist and kind person. If Dr. Kraemer ignited my interest in the science of exercise and nutrition, then Richard Feinman, PhD, poured gasoline on the flame. He has one of the greatest scientific minds in nutrition, and our countless intellectual discussions have challenged almost everything I thought I knew about nutrition and science. Maria Luz Fernandez, PhD, has gone above and beyond as a friend and colleague supporting and enhancing all my current research and Stephen Phinney, MD, PhD, is a true genius who has provided invaluable guidance and support.

It is also necessary to acknowledge another critical person that had great vision, perseverance, and willingness to challenge the conventional dogma of the time at the expense of ridicule. That person is Dr. Robert C. Atkins. He was a tremendous person who had a remarkable and permanent impact on my life. His recognition of the importance of science to validate his diet approach and his generosity is a major reason I am in a position to write this book. The true impact of his visionary efforts will reach levels beyond even his expectations, as ongoing and future research continues to bring scientific support to the concepts for which he had such ingenious foresight so many years ago.

Last, and of course not least, I am forever grateful to my selfless mother, Nina, and my father, Jerry, for their unconditional love and support, and all the sacrifices they have made in order to make my life better. Finally, I need to thank my wonderful wife, Ana, who keeps me balanced and makes life infinitely more fun.

—J.V.

TRANSFORM YOUR BODY— AND YOUR LIFE

At the risk of sounding like an infomercial, what if we told you there was a shortcut to achieving the body you want? One that requires only about 90 minutes of exercise a week and doesn't involve calorie counting or depriving yourself of the foods you love? Not only will it help you build a lean, muscular, fit-looking physique, it'll keep you healthy for life, too. Sound good?

Well, the shortcut does exist, and it's what we call the TNT Diet. Of course, more than likely, you've heard a similar spiel before—and so have we. After all, you'll find this type of claim from just about every diet and exercise book on Amazon.com. So what sets TNT apart from the rest? Or, perhaps more accurately, what makes it better? In a word: science.

You see, we didn't just create TNT out of thin air. Or base it on the type of diet that we thought would sell the most books. We also didn't try to take what works for a bodybuilder or professional athlete and adapt it for everyone. (Are *you* a bodybuilder or professional athlete?)

Instead we took a systematic approach, applying cutting-edge nutrition and exercise science to the goals and lifestyles that match those of *most* men. Think of it as working backward: Instead of making your life fit our plan, we've designed our plan to fit your life.

That's because, like you, we live in a world of high-pressure jobs, long commutes, and family responsibilities that demand more and more of our time and energy. All of which leaves little room for exercise. And when it comes to our diets, we recognized the need for a simple, effective approach— not one that turns eating into a hassle. By taking all of these factors into consideration, we tapped into the latest science to create a program that yields the most dramatic results in the least amount of time. And we can prove it. In fact, we already have.

We've scientifically tested TNT—on men (and women) just like you at the University of Connecticut. The results, which we'll share with you throughout this book, are amazing.

For instance, in just 12 weeks, one of the men who participated in our study, Jaimen Sanders (page 53) lost 30 pounds of fat and gained 9 pounds of muscle. Another, Lucas Hutchinson (page 23), dropped 19 pounds of fat and packed on 12 pounds of muscle. Like everyone who follows the TNT Diet, Jaimen and Lucas ate as much as they wanted and exercised just 3 days a week.

These are just a couple of the real-world results that let us know we were on to something revolutionary with TNT. They show the power that this plan has to dramatically remodel *any* body, including yours.

You can harness this power by fully committing to the TNT Diet for a solid 12 weeks. This time frame provides you with the opportunity to experience all of the benefits that TNT has to offer. Based on results from our lab, stick with the plan for 12 weeks, and you can expect to lose 15 to 30 pounds of fat, build several pounds of new muscle, and significantly reduce your risk for heart disease and diabetes. Think of it as an 84-day investment in yourself: The payoff is huge, and we can't think of one downside—except that you'll probably need to buy all new clothes. And, hey, you could probably use a style upgrade anyway.

TNT is a practical diet and exercise program that leverages the latest science to make your life easier and healthier. We'll show you the data and explain how, by following a few simple guidelines, you can enjoy the same success as those who've already participated in the program.

Before we get to all that, though, we'll try to anticipate a few of your initial questions.

WHO ARE YOU GUYS?

This is an important question, since just about every expert has a bunch of letters after his or her name. And besides showing that you've managed to master academia, those letters don't necessarily mean anything—except that you're probably still paying off school loans. But my coauthor, Jeff Volek, PhD, RD, an associate professor of kinesiology and registered dietitian at the University of Connecticut, is one expert who lives up to his credentials.

During the last decade, Jeff has authored or coauthored more than 140 scientific papers on diet and exercise, and has conducted more studies on low-carbohydrate diets than any other researcher in the world. He was also trained by—and still works closely with—William Kraemer, PhD, who is widely recognized as the most influential muscle and strength researcher in history. You should know that Jeff doesn't just write about his research, he actually uses it. Case in point: In 2000, he won the Indiana state power-lifting championship in the 181-pound weight class with a body-fat percentage of less than 10 percent. The highlights of his victory were a 315-pound bench press, a 585-pound squat, and a 600-pound deadlift.

As for me, I'm Adam Campbell, the features editor of *Men's Health* magazine. I make my living as a journalist, but I also have a master's degree in exercise physiology, and I'm a National Strength and Conditioning Association (NSCA) certified strength and conditioning specialist (CSCS). My job, practically my whole life, revolves around helping guys like you find the best ways to eat and exercise for fat loss, muscle gain, and better health. So over the years, I've interviewed and worked with hundreds of fitness and nutrition experts, read thousands of studies, and spent a good deal of time studying anatomy and physiology textbooks. Through all of this, I began to notice how most of the mainstream diet and exercise recommendations actually contradict scientific logic. In fact, the typical advice that's given to the American public doesn't mesh with what the *best* scientists, trainers, and dietitians advise either. Which is probably the reason so many people are frustrated with the way they look and feel.

And that's why Jeff and I teamed up to create TNT. Our objective: to design a program that combines the science of fat loss and muscle growth with the realities of everyday, 21st-century life. All in order to give you the power to transform your body without having to restructure your life.

. . . AND WHAT EXACTLY IS TNT?

TNT, or Targeted Nutrition Tactics, is just what it sounds like: specific nutrition (and exercise) strategies that enable you to reach your body composition goals as fast as possible. Notice that we purposely used the term *body composition,* instead of *weight loss.* Sure, it's a bit geeky, but it also makes a lot of sense. The reason is that, *technically,* TNT isn't a weight-loss plan.

You see, we started this book with the basic assumption that pretty much no one likes body fat. So our first task was to create a plan that maximizes fat loss, without sacrificing muscle. After all, what guy wants to lose even one muscle fiber? Trouble is, that's what happens on almost all diets, especially those that don't include weight training. In fact, for every 10 pounds that a person loses on a typical diet, 2 to 3 of those are from muscle. And that's why TNT is focused on body *composition,* not body *weight.*

A brief explanation: *Body composition* is a term that essentially describes your body's ratio of fat to muscle, otherwise known as your *body-fat percentage.* For instance, if you lose 7 pounds of fat and 3 pounds of muscle, your scale shows a 10-pound weight loss. But had you simply dropped the 7 pounds of fat, without the muscle loss, your body-fat percentage would be lower, even though you'd actually weigh more.

That said, TNT will allow you to lose all the weight you want. And you'll lose it faster than you would with other approaches. But it will be what we call *quality* weight loss. In other words, the weight you lose will be pure fat, instead of fat *and* muscle. And the result will be a dramatic improvement in your body composition.

But there's more to TNT than simply losing fat. That's because it can be customized for *anyone's* goals. In fact, you can use TNT to build muscle and lose fat *simultaneously*—a feat that most nutrition and fitness experts will tell you is impossible. Yet by using the scientific principles of metabolism and physiology, we've created a plan that will help you do just that. As a result, TNT not only works for the guy who wants to lose 50 pounds of fat, but also for the guy who wants to trade 10 pounds of fat for 10 pounds of muscle.

WHAT WILL I EAT?

TNT is all about eating the right foods at the right times. Starting in Chapter 1, you'll quickly learn that the foundation of the plan is a low-carbohydrate diet—or what we think of as a meat-and-vegetables diet. An example of dinner might be a large rib-eye steak with steamed broccoli and butter, a meal that's hardly tantamount to typical diet food.

Along the way, you'll also find out how and when you can eat carbohydrates—such as bread, pasta, and rice—in order to build muscle without gaining fat. For instance, this is when you might have spaghetti and meatballs with French bread. So depending on your body composition goals, you'll be able to eat a wide variety of foods—the key is simply making sure you eat them at the appropriate times.

Rather than promote moderation—which results in slow and often disappointing progress—we put an emphasis on the extremes in nutrient composition. This doesn't mean *extreme dieting*—which, in our view, is a phrase that describes a low-calorie diet. It simply means that you'll choose specific foods at specific times of the day or week. So *extremes in nutrient composition* simply refers to the amount of fat and carbohydrates in any given meal. In general, when fat is high, carbohydrates will be low; when carbohydrates are high, fat will be low. You can compare this to smart play-calling in football. If you have a strong running game (meat and vegetables), then mixing in a few well-timed play-action passes (bread, pasta, rice) will often lead to big gains. TNT takes the same approach with your diet, only instead of touchdowns, your gains will come in the form of new muscle. Don't worry; it's not complicated once you understand the general guidelines of our plan.

Of course, most popular diet books these days promote an "all things in moderation" philosophy. And if this type of strategy works for you, we highly recommend it. After all, if you can eat anything you want, avoid overeating, and build the body you want while lowering your risk for disease, then why not do that? But we've found that for the moderate approach to work effectively, it typically requires paying close attention to your calorie intake, and more often than not, the improvements in body composition are mediocre.

Compared to these conventional diets, our "extreme" eating plan causes the body to adapt in a more robust manner, which is the key to simultaneously gaining muscle and losing fat. Think of it this way: *Extreme* is another way of saying "beyond the average," or "extraordinary." So if you want extreme results, it only makes sense to follow an extreme diet.

WHAT KIND OF EXERCISE WILL I DO?

The answer here is simple: weight training. Why? Because it's not only the best mode of exercise for building and maintaining muscle, it's also the best for elevating your metabolism and torching fat. (You'll find out why, of course.) All of which make it the most efficient form of training you can do.

Just like the diet, the TNT Workout Plan has been designed to help you achieve the best results in the least amount of time. It's based on 50 years of muscle research and the lessons we've learned in our lab, as well as those from interviewing and working with hundreds of strength coaches, bodybuilders, and personal trainers over the past decade.

As a result, the workouts are fast and effective. Which is why you'll only be required to exercise 3 days a week, for about 30 minutes at a time. That's long enough to complete a highly effective fat-burning, muscle-building workout, but short enough to change your clothes, hit the gym, and shower, without needing more than a lunch hour.

WHAT ABOUT MY HEALTH?

This isn't a book about vanity. Sure, looking better may be an important motivator for you. But the impact of TNT extends far beyond the reflection you see in the mirror. In fact, it's not a leap to suggest that it will help you dramatically improve your entire life.

Your health.

Your relationships.

Your career.

Even your future.

You may think this is hyperbole, but we've seen it firsthand in hundreds of men and women. And we've experienced it for ourselves. The truth is, even though the promise of a lean midsection may be your reason for buying this book, you may soon find that it simply becomes an ancillary benefit.

We've spent years studying how food and exercise affect the human body. Not just in terms of weight loss, but also muscle growth, physical and mental performance, mood, energy levels, and the aging process. We've also examined the impact of food and exercise on the risk for heart disease, diabetes, and cancer. And, it turns out, all of these factors are highly interconnected. Intuitively, of course, this makes sense: A truly healthy diet and exercise plan should enhance every aspect of your overall well-being. Only most guys don't think of it that way. That might very well be why the majority of men who start a diet end up abandoning it within 6 months, if not sooner.

So we have a simple request when you start TNT: Give it a fair shot, and follow the plan for an entire 12 weeks. Along the way, pay close attention to your body. Not just the visible transformation, but the changes that are occurring on the inside. For instance, the ones your doctor sees when he examines your blood work; the kind your better half notices because you're in a better mood; and those you discover yourself, when you suddenly realize you're sleeping better, you have more energy, and your work productivity has improved.

Of course, you'll never know all of this if you take a halfhearted approach to our plan. But follow through with it—from day 1 to day 84—and you may find that it changes your life forever. Beyond the science, we can tell you that the TNT Diet is exactly what we follow ourselves and that it has had a tremendous impact on both of our lives. Which is precisely the reason we wanted to share it with you.

DOES IT WORK FOR WOMEN?

Absolutely. But because one of the driving principles of our plan is that you maintain and even build muscle while you lose weight, women are sometimes hesitant to jump on board. Especially since it requires lifting weights. This is simply based on the fear of "getting big," which most women have an aversion to, even if it's muscle and not fat.

However, we've studied the effect of resistance training on women for several years now, and the women we've worked with experienced only desirable changes to their figures. The main reason is that women aren't genetically engineered to increase their muscle mass significantly. The fact is, they have a limited capacity to produce testosterone, the hormone that's responsible for controlling the rate at which your body builds muscle. So trust us when we say that women don't have to worry about adding an impressive amount of muscle.

Now, if you're a woman, and you start our plan, you may feel like your muscles are getting bigger right away. But there are a couple of key points to remember: First, you may experience some slight swelling initially because you'll be working your muscles in ways you never have before. The swelling won't be visible to the naked eye, but you might notice it by feel. You'll also be more aware of your muscles. If you've never lifted before, you'll probably find that it feels good, but that it also makes you think about your muscles more often. This can lead to the perception that they're growing.

That said, most women could stand to gain a little muscle anyway. Muscle burns fat—so the more you have, the greater your ability to flatten your belly and melt away your hips. Plus, muscle takes up less space than fat, which means that even if you gain a little muscle as you lose fat, you'll still be getting smaller.

The bottom line: Pay close attention to how your clothes fit, especially those tight-fitting jeans. In no time, you'll find they're fitting better than ever. So let that—and the mirror—be your main guide.

OPEN YOUR MIND, RESULTS WILL FOLLOW

It might surprise you to know we were hesitant to write this book. The diet and fitness industry is so full of conflicting information that it's become nearly impossible for most folks to know who to trust. For instance, one expert says to eat a low-fat diet, while another says to eat low-carb. And then, of course, there's a third who claims that both approaches are wrong, and a fourth who says everyone's right.

So how do you know who to believe? Is it the MD or the PhD? The doctor you most often see on TV? Maybe it's the expert who promotes a plan that best fits what you've always been told. It could be that you're so confused you don't bother with any of it.

We get it. And frankly, we don't blame you. But that's why we based the TNT Diet entirely on science—not myths, flawed logic, and unproven trends. It's also why we wanted to share this science with you throughout the pages of this book, instead of simply saying, "Eat this way." After all, your body is your most important asset; you should understand all of the details behind our recommendations.

Read the chapters that follow with an open mind, and you'll quickly see how much of what you've been told about diet and exercise is flat-out wrong, or at the very least misguided. More importantly, though, you'll learn a new, more effective and more efficient method for permanently transforming your body—and improving your life.

—**Adam Campbell**

TNT TRANSFORMATION

"My waistline shrunk, and I could see my muscles again."

Name: **Keith Ayotte**
Age: **23**
Height: **5 feet 9 inches**
Weight before: **260**
Weight after: **225**

WHEN WE ASKED KEITH AYOTTE why he decided to try TNT, his answer couldn't have been clearer: "I was sick of being overweight."

For most of his life, though, carrying around excess baggage had actually been unfamiliar territory to Keith: "Growing up, I was a football player and a speed skater, which helped automatically keep me lean." Unfortunately, all that changed when he arrived at college. "I quit being active and ate whatever I wanted," he says. "As a result, I gained 70 pounds."

Soon after, Keith discovered the TNT Diet study we were conducting at the University of Connecticut and quickly signed up for it. His experience echoes what we hear from almost everyone: "The first 4 days I was tired, but after 2 weeks, I was energetic all day long," he says. "And to think, before I started, I would often fall asleep in the middle of the day."

In our 12-week study, Keith added 50 pounds to his bench press while losing a whopping 35 pounds. Even more impressive was his improvement in risk for heart disease. He lowered his blood pressure from 130/98 to 110/72. His total cholesterol dropped 30 percent, and his triglycerides plummeted a staggering 61 percent. But the improvements in his personal life may have been even more impressive: "My girlfriend not only said that I looked sexier, but that I was also in a better mood and far less grumpy." Now think about this: If your significant other could say the same thing about you, how much better might your relationship be?

PART I: THE BASICS

CHAPTER 1

DON'T BELIEVE EVERYTHING YOU READ

There's a precise, if seemingly contradictory, way to describe the average guy: skinny-fat. Of course, you might think "fat-fat," or simply "fat," apply better to what you see in the mirror. But chances are, the word "skinny" is quite relevant, too.

Why? Because most men lose muscle with every passing year. So even though you may not *look* skinny, technically you are—at least when it comes to your muscle.

Case in point: Without even realizing it, the average guy loses 6 pounds of muscle between the ages of 30 and 50. For perspective, that's about the same amount of muscle on your right arm.

Now keep in mind, muscle doesn't turn to fat. But lose it, and it will likely be *replaced* by fat over time, according to a study in the *American Journal of Clinical Nutrition*. Trading muscle for fat not only makes you look flabby, but it also increases your pant size—even if you somehow manage to keep your scale weight the same. The reason: Each pound of fat takes up 18 percent more space in your body than each pound of muscle.

It gets worse: Fat cells secrete hormones that signal your body to break down muscle tissue. So the more fat you gain, the greater your risk for muscle loss over time. All of which creates a perpetual cycle that leads to even more fat and less muscle. The end result: skinny-fat.

This also helps explain why weight gain seems to sneak up on so many people. Sure, it may sometimes feel like it happens overnight, but adding notches to your belt usually occurs over time. Our colleagues at the University of Connecticut determined that men, on average, gain about a pound of body weight annually from ages 25 to 45. See the problem? An extra pound each year is hardly noticeable on a month-to-month basis, but one day, you suddenly realize that you're carrying around 20 more pounds of flab than you did in high school.

So why does this now seem to be the norm, despite the fact that most Americans are more health conscious than ever? The simple answer is that the way you've been taught to eat and exercise is nearly the exact opposite of what science actually shows to be most effective—for both losing fat *and* building muscle. And this really shouldn't be surprising. The majority of health and nutrition experts—yes, even those you see on television—promote methods that aren't supported by scientific research, or even by the most basic laws of human metabolism and physiology. But to fully understand the reason, we'll first need to introduce you to glycogen.

THE SECRET REASON YOU'RE FAT

Glycogen is the name for carbohydrates that are stored in your muscles. An easy way to understand glycogen is to picture it as a storage tank for sugar, the form of carbohydrate your body uses for fuel. So just as you have fat stores, you also have sugar stores. However, unlike your fat stores, which are able to expand (read: you can get fatter and fatter), your glycogen tank has a limited capacity to store sugar. For instance, think of your car: If you own a midsize, you probably have about a 14-gallon fuel tank. Try to fill it with 20 gallons, though, and the other 6 would spill out onto the pavement. It's the same way with sugar and your glycogen tank.

And therein lies the problem: A full glycogen tank signals your body to use incoming carbohydrates for energy instead of your stored fat. Otherwise, your glycogen tank will overflow. As a result, your body not only stops burning fat, it starts conserving it—just in case of starvation. This is one of the main reasons for America's growing obesity problem. Because most people's diets are excessively high in carbohydrates, their glycogen levels are always at peak capacity. In turn, their bodies won't allow them to use their stored fat for energy.

What's more, there are also serious health ramifications to perpetually high glycogen levels. When excess carbohydrates from your diet can't be stored as sugar in your glycogen tank, the overflow causes sugar to build up in your bloodstream. The result: chronically high blood sugar, which can damage the large blood vessels of your heart and brain, and the small vessels of your kidneys and eyes. As a consequence, your body starts shuttling the overflow of sugar to your liver, where it's then converted to a blood fat known as *triglycerides*. If you've ever had blood work done, you might recognize triglycerides as one of the measurements that your doctor ordered. And for good reason: Elevated triglycerides are a risk factor for heart disease and an early predictor of future diabetes. To make matters even worse, once sugar becomes triglycerides, or fat, it can be stored as fat. Ever been told carbs can't make you fat? Think again.

Now, there are probably lots of reasons why people have gotten so far off track—the misinterpretation of data from nutrition and exercise studies, valid scientific research that's been ignored or dismissed, the influence of politics and special interest groups, and, in some cases, just good intentions gone bad. But the key to getting back on course is understanding exactly *why* much of what you've been told about diet and exercise is wrong. And your re-education starts now.

You've Been Told: "Follow the Food Guide Pyramid."

The Origin: In 1980, the United States Department of Agriculture (USDA) published its first set of dietary guidelines for Americans, which recommended a carbohydrate-based diet. And, in an effort to make the guidelines easier for the public to understand, they released the original Food Guide Pyramid in 1992. As a general rule of thumb, people were told to consume six or more servings of grain products—bread, cereals, pasta, and rice—each day. These are essentially the same recommendations that we are given to this day.

What Science Shows: If you look at dietary intake in the United States over the last three decades from the National Health and Nutrition Examination Surveys (NHANES), you'll notice an interesting pattern. In men, average daily energy intake during the early 1970s was 2,450 calories. But by the year 2000, that number had increased to 2,618. An even greater increase in calories was seen in women. Where did these extra calories come from? According to the NHANES data, it was almost exclusively derived from carbohydrates. Interestingly, there were minuscule changes in the intake of protein and fat.

So sure, people are eating too much. But they're eating too many carbohydrates, not too much protein and fat. And that's a glaring problem with the government's nutrition recommendations—one that's seemingly being ignored. For example, in 2005, the USDA unveiled a new food guide pyramid, now called MyPyramid. Despite the steep rise in obesity with the previous guidelines in place, there were very few changes made to the pyramid's overall philosophy. (See "A Pyramid Scam?")

You've Been Told: "Always exercise in the fat-burning zone."

The Origin: In 1993, University of Texas researchers determined that you burn a greater percentage of calories from fat during light- to moderate-intensity exercise than you do when you exercise at a high intensity. In fact, the rate your body burns fat peaks at about 65 percent of your aerobic capacity. For most people, that's equivalent to a walk or jog in which your effort is

---

A Pyramid Scam?

When MyPyramid (www.mypyramid.gov) was released in 2005, it was applauded for two reasons: First, because it included the "revolutionary" recommendation to exercise. And second, the pyramid could now be customized to suit a person's body type and level of activity.

This actually sounds useful, and a step in the right direction, but let's see what kind of information the customizable food pyramid provides us with. Since the average American male is about 31 years old, 5 feet 9 inches, and 180 pounds, we entered those numbers into the MyPyramid calculator, which can be found on its Web site. Then, for activity level, we chose less than 30 minutes a day, since that's most representative as well. According to MyPyramid's computation, the average American man needs eight servings of grains a day. To put that in perspective, that's the equivalent of eight slices of bread or 8 cups of, say, Cheerios. That's a lot of carbohydrates, and ask any expert what the main (and really only) function of carbs in your diet is, and he or she will correctly say, "to provide energy." But now consider: Isn't reducing energy precisely what most people need to do in order to lose weight? The logic doesn't jibe. This is the first indication of exactly how "unfit" the MyPyramid actually is. After all, does anyone really need eight slices of bread a day? Of course not. In fact, we'd suggest that if you want to keep your glycogen levels topped off, the USDA is telling you exactly how to do it.

such that you can still talk easily. Exercise harder than that, though, and the percentage of calories you burn from fat goes down, while the percentage of calories burned from carbs goes up—it's a sliding scale. This finding was appealing because it seemed to suggest that easier exercise—for instance, a slow jog—was more effective at burning fat than harder exercise, such as vigorous weight training or 400-meter sprints.

What Science Shows: You lose fat faster by exercising in the *carb*-burning zone. This is when you're exercising hard, often going nearly all out for 30 to 60 seconds at a time. There are two reasons for this. The first is that even though you burn a lower percentage of fat during this type of high-intensity exercise, the *total* amount of fat you burn is similar to that of light and moderate activity. That's because the harder you go, the more calories per minute you burn. So even though the percentage of fat you burn is smaller, it's in relation to a bigger number of total calories. Think of Kobe Bryant on a poor shooting night: He may only hit 35 percent of his shots, but he'll often launch enough jumpers to still be the game's leading scorer.

The second reason: If you primarily burn fat during exercise, you're automatically burning fewer carbohydrates. That means you're not significantly reducing your glycogen levels. And this diminishes your ability to burn fat when you're not exercising. However, exercise in the carb-burning zone, and you'll deplete your glycogen tank. This will allow you to burn more fat while you're sitting at your desk and lounging on your couch.

The upshot is that the harder you exercise, the more glycogen you burn. Interestingly, German researchers reported this very same finding in 1934. So this isn't new science. It's just a better interpretation of the science as it relates to fat loss.

You've Been Told: "Fat makes you fat."

The Origin: Years ago, in an effort to help people control their weight, government health officials and nutritionists recommended a simple solution: Cut back on fat. And in 1990, they put a number on it, recommending that fat should make up no more than 30 percent of a person's total daily calories. From a mathematical perspective, it seemed logical: Both carbohydrates and protein contain about 4 calories per gram; fat contains about 9 calories per gram. So the theory was that decreasing fat intake would lead to a greater reduction in calories than cutting back on the same amount of carbs. But over time, the message simply became, "Fat makes you fat."

What Science Shows: Fat, itself, doesn't make you fat. For example, in our lab at the University of Connecticut, we've shown that people who eat 60 to 70 percent of their calories from fat lose weight faster than those who eat just 20 percent of their calories from fat.

Of course, eating an overabundance of calories—from fat or anything else—*will* make you fat. So although the original idea to limit fat intake might have made sense on paper, it mistakenly assumed that people wouldn't replace fat calories with even more calories from glycogen-filling carbohydrates. In fact, a 2002 review from the USDA Human Nutrition Research Center at Tufts University found that consuming highly processed carbohydrates such as white bread, pasta, and rice, as well as sugar—approved staples of traditional guidelines for a low-fat diet—promotes an increase in total calorie consumption. And don't forget that the calories that have been added to the daily American diet since the 1970s were almost entirely composed of carbohydrates.

One reason for this failed experiment: Fat is a powerful satiator, keeping you satisfied for a longer period of time after you eat than carbohydrates. So it's likely that as your fat intake is reduced, and replaced with carbs, your hunger will increase.

Another important factor: Carbohydrates raise your blood levels of insulin, a powerful hormone that stimulates your body to stop burning—and start storing—fat. So when you eat lots of carbohydrates—as the typical American does, or as you would on a low-fat diet—your ability to burn fat is inhibited, impairing fat loss. On the other hand, low-carb diets, which are high in fat, keep your insulin levels low, allowing your body to break down stored fat for energy.

You've Been Told: "Eat carbs for energy."

The Origin: In the 1960s, researchers demonstrated the importance of glycogen as a fuel for high-level athletes during prolonged exercise—such as long-distance running. For instance, the scientists determined that high glycogen levels were associated with better endurance performance than low glycogen levels. As a result, elite athletes were encouraged to eat lots of carbohydrates after they worked out, in order to replenish glycogen for the next day's training session or competition. The idea, of course, was to ensure optimal performance. And eventually, this advice trickled down to the average Joe.

What Science Shows: Although it's true that glycogen can be an important fuel source for peak athletic performance, emerging research is challenging the theory that it's merely a storage form of carbohydrate. That's because, as we've touched on briefly, the level of your glycogen tank has a major impact on your ability to burn fat and on your metabolic health. We'll delve into the science fully in Chapter 2, but the important point is this: What helps a world-class marathoner run faster has nothing to do with helping the average guy lose fat. After all, Olympic marathoners burn several thousand calories a day. So unless you exercise like an athlete, eating like an athlete simply doesn't apply.

That's not to say that consuming the right amount of carbohydrates after your workout can't have benefits—it can. And we'll explain exactly how throughout the course of this book. However, stockpiling carbs is extremely misguided advice for the average person who consumes the typical American diet.

You've Been Told: "Fat-free foods are good for you."

The Origin: For most of the last three decades, major health organizations such as the American Heart Association and the American Diabetes Association have warned that consuming fat, and particularly saturated fat, raises your risk for heart disease. As a result, fat phobia swept the nation, and even those who weren't dieting started to avoid fat for fear of "clogged arteries." This also created a grand opportunity for the food industry: new product categories, such as fat-free, low-fat, and reduced-fat foods.

What Science Shows: The connection between fat, even saturated fat, and heart disease has never actually been demonstrated. (See Chapter 13 for a complete explanation.) In fact, research from our lab as well as many others shows that replacing carbohydrates with fat—any type of fat, including saturated—actually *lowers* your risk for cardiovascular disease. As a result, even the highly conservative American Heart Association no longer suggests an upper limit for total fat intake, only for that of saturated fat. Yet fat-free and low-fat foods have remained staples of the American diet.

Why? Because the idea that fat is evil has become entrenched in the average person's psyche. If that describes you, consider this logic:

1. Fat-free foods are healthy.

2. Skittles are fat-free.

3. Therefore, Skittles are healthy.

Make sense? Of course not. But it's exactly the type of reasoning that food manufacturers want you to use.

You see, in our example, we started with a false premise. That's because the term *fat-free* is often code for *high-sugar*—an attribute that makes a product the opposite of healthy. For instance, Johns Hopkins University researchers recently determined that high blood sugar is an independent risk factor for heart disease. So high-glycemic foods—those such as sugars and starches that raise your blood sugar dramatically—are inherently unhealthy when eaten all the time. Of course, the other effect of high-sugar foods is that they replenish your glycogen stores and raise your insulin levels, both of which inhibit your ability to burn fat.

Unfortunately, many food manufacturers depend on the success of faulty food logic. After all, lots of people assume that if a food is "healthy" or "fat free" then it won't cause weight gain. So they'll be more likely to indulge in, say, low-fat potato chips than the regular version, even though the former contains more glycogen-filling carbohydrates. (Manufacturers typically remove fat only to replace it with carbs, often in the form of sugar.) In fact, Cornell University researchers reported that when overweight men and women thought they were eating low-fat M&Ms, they consumed 47 percent more calories than those who were given regular M&Ms. The kicker: The only difference between the candies was the label—they were all regular M&Ms. The scientists also determined that, on average, low-fat foods contain 59 percent less fat, but only 15 percent fewer calories than full-fat products.

You've Been Told: "Running is the best way to lose weight."

The Origin: In 1977, Jim Fixx published *The Complete Book of Running.* This best-selling book popularized the notion of running to improve health and lose weight, and is widely credited with kicking off the jogging boom of the 1980s. Furthermore, most exercise scientists during this time were recreational or competitive runners themselves. As a result, running and other types of endurance activities were the type of exercise that was most often studied, particularly in terms of health benefits (and there are many).

And because these researchers reported that running burns a lot more calories than weight training—while requiring nothing but a pair of functional legs—the majority of experts began to widely promote it as the best mode of exercise for fat loss. However, they didn't—and still don't—have the data to support that assertion.

What Science Shows: First, it's important to point out that engaging in a regular running program, or any kind of exercise for that matter, without also adopting a prudent diet is a very inefficient way to lose

The Corporate Fatness Center

We're not sure, but we think we coined this term—and it's certainly relevant. Working long hours in an office setting is a major contributor to the modern male's ever-expanding waistline and shrinking muscles. For instance, a recent Australian study of 1,579 people found that men whose jobs require more than 6 hours of chair time a day are 68 percent more likely to wind up overweight than those who sit less. And University of North Carolina–Wilmington researchers discovered that, on average, people gain 17 pounds within 8 months of starting a sedentary office job.

Which, of course, is why health clubs were invented. Trouble is, only 19 percent of men regularly perform high levels of physical activity outside of work, according to the National Center for Health Statistics. What's more, Norwegian scientists determined that people with the highest job demands had the worst exercise habits. So all of this, combined with a high-carb diet, means you never have to dip into your glycogen tank. As a result, your body burns as little fat as possible.

Don't worry, though: By instituting the principles of the TNT Diet, you'll be able lose your gut for good—and without having to quit your day job.

weight. After all, a typical fast-food double-decker cheeseburger and large fries contain more than 1,100 calories—a meal most red-blooded American men can wolf down in less than 5 minutes. However, to *burn* that many calories, the average guy would have to run for 53 minutes at an 8½-minute-per-mile pace. Which is why your diet has a greater impact on total weight loss than exercise.

As we've already discussed, though, it's not simply weight loss that's important—it's the quality of your weight loss that matters most. That is, the amount of your weight loss that's pure fat, since that's what really counts. Perhaps surprisingly, endurance exercise—such as running, cycling, or walking—does little to further augment *fat* loss when combined with a good diet. Weight training, however, has a dramatic impact. Consider a study we conducted back in 1999. We put overweight men on a diet that was approximately 1,500 calories a day, and then divided them into either a diet-only group, a diet group that also performed endurance exercise, or a diet group that performed both endurance exercise and weight training.

After 3 months, men in each of the groups had lost almost the same amount of weight—about 21 pounds. But the quality of their weight loss was much different. The men in the weight-training group lost 5 pounds more fat than the other two groups. You might wonder how that's possible when they all dropped the same amount of weight. The answer is that the men who dieted or dieted and performed only endurance exercise lost about 15 pounds of fat, but also lost several pounds of muscle. Those who lifted weights lost almost pure fat.

You see, weight training is a powerful tool when it comes to fat loss. Because it stimulates your muscles to grow, your body is less apt to part with your hard-earned muscle. This is crucial because the more muscle you have, the bigger your body's fat-burning furnace. What's more, if you lose muscle, you not only reduce your ability to burn fat, your glycogen tank becomes smaller. (Remember, most of your glycogen is located in your muscles.) So you have less room to store carbohydrates, increasing the likelihood that they'll be converted to fat in your liver. Endurance exercise provides none of these benefits.

But what about the fact that running burns more calories than weight training? Turns out, when scientists at the University of Southern Maine used an advanced method to estimate energy expenditure during exercise, they found that weight training burns as many as 71 percent more calories than originally thought. In fact, the researchers calculated that performing just one circuit of eight exercises—which takes about 8 minutes—can expend 159 to 231 calories. That's about the same as running at a 6-minute-per-mile pace for the same duration. And just as important, research shows that weight training, unlike endurance exercise, can elevate your metabolism for up to 39 hours after your workout session.

HOW TO LOSE YOUR GUT FOR GOOD

If you've been paying attention, you already know the answer: Use the opposite approach to what you've been accustomed to. That means taking measures—read: the right diet and exercise program—to reduce glycogen. This triggers your body to start using fat as its primary source of energy, accelerating the rate at which you lose belly flab. In fact, it's scientifically proven that this strategy preferentially reduces abdominal fat in men. Even better, it helps to spark nutrient partitioning, an effect that allows you to simultaneously burn fat and build muscle. Ready to find out how? Turn the page.

"No, I'm not taking steroids!"

Name: Keith Suthammanont
Age: 21
Height: 5 feet 9 inches
Weight before: 185
Weight after: 165

AS KEITH SUTHAMMANONT KNOWS, the truth can hurt—but sometimes it's exactly what you need to hear. "When I was 18, I showed up to a family function wearing a form-fitting shirt, and one of my aunts said, 'I guess you're going to be the chubby brother,'" says Keith. "This lit a fire under me because, for her to say something, I must have really let myself go."

As a result, Keith decided to give TNT a shot. In a matter of weeks, he lost 20 pounds of fat, and sculpted his skinny-fat physique into a defined, muscular body. The speed of his results didn't go unnoticed. "Following my weight loss, people starting asking me how I did it," he says. "And from time to time, I'd even get accused of taking steroids! While that was frustrating, it was also flattering, because I realized that people were really noticing the changes I'd made."

Three years after his physical transformation, TNT is still having a major impact on Keith's life: The experience he had improving his own health and fitness inspired him to help others do the same. As a result, Keith now makes his living as a personal trainer. And we say every client he has is lucky: After all, who better to learn from than a guy who's been where you are, and has gotten to where you want to be?

CHAPTER 2

TRADE YOUR BELLY FOR BICEPS

A lmost all men say that their number one fitness goal is to "lose fat and build muscle." And while that's no surprise, many scientists, personal trainers, and dietitians claim that those are actually separate goals—that you can't accomplish both simultaneously.

Why? Because there's a widely held belief among these experts that your body won't allow you to gain a significant amount of muscle without also adding fat. At the same time, such experts will tell you that you'd be hard-pressed to lose fat without sacrificing some of your muscle. For instance, research on dieters shows that, on average, 75 percent of their weight loss is fat, and 25 percent is muscle. So you have to choose one goal or the other, these experts say. To which we offer a simple reply: Hogwash.

The problem is that the vast majority of fitness and nutrition experts subscribe to an approach that focuses mainly on the number of calories you consume. Want to gain muscle? You'll need to eat more calories than you burn—even though that means that you'll also pack on fat. Weight loss your goal? Do the opposite, but be prepared to part with some of your hard-earned muscle. So no matter what you decide, it's a win-lose proposition. The idea is that, at any one time, your body can only be growing bigger—by building new muscle and adding to your fat stores—or getting smaller, by breaking down muscle and fat for energy. This concept is so well established as "fact" that even we used to think this way ourselves.

But imagine, for a moment, if you had the power to control what your body does with the calories you eat. For example, instead of storing your calories as belly flab, you'd turn them into sleeve-busting muscle. And because you'd be using those incoming nutrients to build more-muscular arms, you'd automatically burn your stored fat for energy. Think of it as the panacea for the modern male body: Your biceps grow as your love handles shrink.

WHAT YOU CAN LEARN FROM A PIG

All your life, you've been trained to think in terms of calories. Which, of course, is useful. But we want you to adopt a slightly different mindset: Instead of concentrating on the number of calories you consume, start focusing on where those calories go. This is a concept known as *nutrient partitioning*. And it's the key to creating the metabolic shift that allows you to simultaneously build muscle and lose fat. That's because nutrient partitioning refers to the process in which calories are diverted away from your fat cells and redirected toward your muscle cells. (It works in reverse, too.)

If you've never heard of this, you might wonder if it's even possible. So let's start with a basic, albeit odd, example: Growth hormone–treated pigs. Research shows that when pigs are given growth hormone, their fat stores decrease by 50 to 80 percent, while their muscle mass increases by 10 to 20 percent. Growth hormone treatment accomplishes this by inhibiting certain enzymes that are involved in fat storage, while stimulating other enzymes related to muscle growth. What's more, these effects are seen while the pigs are eating 10 to 15 percent fewer calories than usual. In other words, the pigs eat less, gain more muscle, and lose more fat when they're on growth hormone. Ever notice how lean pork is these days? That's due to nutrient partitioning.

All of which sounds pretty fascinating, but leads to the million-dollar question: Can we create nutrient partitioning in humans? And, just as important, can we do it with diet and exercise, and not drugs? The short answer: Yes.

INSULIN: A DOUBLE-EDGED SWORD

You've already learned that your glycogen levels can dramatically impact the degree to which your body burns fat. If your glycogen tank is full, you'll burn very little fat; if it's depleted, your fat-burning furnace will be turned on high. But how exactly does this work? And what does this have to do with nutrient partitioning and building muscle? The key is a hormone called insulin.

Insulin levels rise whenever your blood sugar rises. That's because insulin's primary duty is to move glucose—the form of sugar your body uses for energy—from your bloodstream into your muscle cells. Once in your muscles, glucose can be burned as fuel or stored as glycogen for later use. This, by the way, is how your body helps prevent dangerously high levels of blood sugar, like the kind associated with type 2 diabetes.

Here's where food enters the picture: Unlike protein and fat—which have little if any impact on blood sugar—carbohydrates such as starch and sugar are quickly broken down into glucose during digestion and absorbed into your bloodstream. Thus, the more carbs you eat, the higher and faster your blood sugar rises. As a result, the higher your insulin levels rise, too.

Why does insulin matter? When your glycogen stores are full, insulin puts both your fat and muscle cells in growth mode. This pretty much guarantees that you won't be burning either for energy. While that's great for your biceps, it's a horrible scenario for your belly. After all, the idea is to deflate your gut, not make it bigger. But remember, insulin's job is to move glucose out of your bloodstream quickly; this is a necessity in order for you to maintain healthy blood sugar levels. So if there's no room in your muscles to store glucose, then your body wants to use up as much of that glucose floating around in your bloodstream for fuel as possible. And that means it doesn't want to provide your muscles with energy from any other source, including the fat from your midsection.

Trouble is, when you eat more carbohydrates than can readily be burned—and your glycogen tank is full—your body has only one choice: Start converting the excess glucose from all those carbs to fat. Glucose is then diverted away from your muscle cells—where glycogen is located—and toward your fat cells. And that's a prime example of nutrient partitioning—even though it's the type that you definitely don't want. The bottom line: When glycogen is at peak capacity, insulin is a double-edged sword. It helps you build muscle—as long as you also provide the right nutrients and type of exercise (keep reading)—but also leads to more fat. Which is why most experts believe you can't build muscle without gaining fat.

FLIPPING YOUR CELLULAR SWITCH

Now for the good news: Low glycogen levels change your body's response to insulin. Insulin still signals your body to build muscle—again, given the right conditions—but it no longer blocks your ability to burn fat. Why? Because your body is smart. It makes refilling your glycogen levels a priority, just in case of an energy emergency. So it sucks any carbs you eat into your muscles to be stored as glycogen. As a result, your body has to turn to fat—the kind you pack around your belly—as its primary fuel source. After all, if your body were to keep burning carbs, it would only be limiting its ability to replenish glycogen. Or to put it in everyday terms, you save money a lot faster when you don't spend it.

At this time, it's like you have an internal traffic cop diverting glucose away from your gut and into your muscles. So your muscle cells are in growth mode, but your fat cells are in breakdown mode. And that means you've created the ideal internal environment for remodeling your body. Think of it as flipping the cellular switch that allows you to burn fat as you build muscle. The next step, then, is to learn how to implement the nutrition and exercise tactics—how to ignite the TNT—that give you complete control over that switch.

TIMING ISN'T EVERYTHING, BUT IT'S CLOSE

These days, it's a popular trend among nutritionists to refer to "good" carbs and "bad" carbs. And while we certainly agree that some sources of carbohydrates are better than others (see Chapter 6), we believe that the total amount of carbs, and when you eat those carbs, are more-important factors to focus on. TNT revolves around the fact that there are "well-timed" carbs and "poorly timed" carbs. Think about it: Eat carbohydrates at the wrong time—for instance, when your glycogen tank is full—and your body stops burning, and starts storing, fat. But eat carbs at the right time—when glycogen levels are low—and those carbs help you build muscle, without increasing the size of your gut. That's why we've based the nutrition tactics in TNT around what we call *Time Zones*. This allows you to know what you should eat, and when you should eat it, in order to customize your diet for your goals. Here, we've summarized each of the Time Zones, but we've provided complete eating guidelines for each Time Zone later in the book.

THE FAT-BURNING TIME ZONE

THE NUTRITION TACTIC: A LOW-CARB DIET
The Benefits
- Speeds Fat Loss
- Reduces Heart Disease Risk
- Regulates Your Appetite

When You'll Use This Tactic: Most of the week. Consider a low-carb diet to be the foundation of the TNT Diet.

What You'll Eat: All of the vegetables, meat, cheese, and eggs that you want. An example of dinner might be a hunk of prime rib served with a Caprese salad of tomatoes, mozzarella, and basil, and topped off with a glass of red wine.

Why It Works: Limiting the number of carbohydrates you con-sume—by filling your plate with protein, fat, and low-starch vegetables—automatically helps you to keep both your glycogen tank and insulin levels low. The result: Your body is always in fat-burning mode, and your risk for heart disease plummets.

This tactic also allows you to eat as much as you desire, without the risk of overeating. For example, in one 6-week study in our lab, men who followed a low-carb diet lost 7 pounds of fat and gained 2 pounds of muscle—all while eating as much food as they wanted. In fact, because our goal in this study was to find out what happens to heart disease risk when you *don't* lose weight on a low-carb diet, we constantly encouraged these guys to eat more. Yet they still experienced a small decrease in body weight. And what's more amazing is that they also gained muscle, even though we didn't ask them to exercise.

THE RELOADING TIME ZONE

THE NUTRITION TACTIC: A HIGH-CARB DIET
The Benefits

- Boosts Muscle Growth
- Instantly Inflates Your Biceps
- Allows You to Eat Pizza

When You'll Use This Tactic: Up to 2 days a week, depend-ing on your goals.

What You'll Eat: Plenty of protein, and lots of carbs, including starchy foods such as bread, pasta, and rice. Although any type of carb is acceptable, we promote the healthiest ones, such as the 100 percent whole grain versions of bread, pasta, and rice, as well as beans, sweet potatoes, yogurt, fruit, and milk.

Why It Works: The carbohydrates you eat will induce a surge of insulin. This surge drives the muscle-building nutrients you gain from downing protein-rich foods right into your muscle cells. It's like your internal traffic cop is not only directing these nutrients toward your pecs, lats, and quads, it's as if he's opened up a couple of more lanes for them to travel.

The downside is that you won't burn fat quite as fast as in the Fat-Burning Time Zone. But because your glycogen levels have been held down by your low-carb diet in the Fat-Burning Time Zone, your muscles will soak up carbohydrates like a sponge, which causes them to feel pumped and look larger almost immediately. This makes it a great strategy to coordinate with a trip to the beach. The trick, of course, is to avoid overeating carbs, which results in an overflowing glycogen tank. That's why we've placed a limit on the total amount of time—about 36 hours at the most—that you can spend in the Reloading Zone.

THE MUSCLE-BUILDING TIME ZONE

THE NUTRITION TACTIC: WORKOUT NUTRITION
The Benefits

- Dramatically Accelerates Muscle Growth
- Speeds Workout Recovery

When You'll Use This Tactic: From 1 hour before you lift weights to 30 minutes after your training session.

What You'll Eat: Depending on your goals (i.e., faster fat loss or more muscle), you'll either eat a snack of protein—such as a protein shake or some tuna—or a snack that contains both protein and carbohydrates, like a turkey sandwich.

Why It Works: Resistance training primes your muscles to grow— all you have to do is feed them. For example, Australian researchers found that men who consumed a protein shake just before and right after their weight workout gained twice as much muscle in 10 weeks as guys who had the same shakes, but downed them at least 5 hours outside of their exercise session.

No matter what your goal, you'll always include protein during this time, since this nutrient provides the raw materials for muscle growth, without inhibiting your body's ability to burn fat. And if you're okay with temporarily slowing fat loss, you can also down a hefty dose of carbohydrates, which will boost muscle growth even more—just as it does in the Reloading Time Zone.

TNT FOR YOUR GOALS

Maybe you have 50, 60, even 100 pounds to lose. Perhaps it's only 10 or 20. Or it might be that you're more interested in packing on serious muscle without packing on lard. Whatever your goal, you can use TNT to achieve it. That's because we've created specific eating strategies based on a range of options. One end of this spectrum is designed to help you achieve maximum fat loss; the other end, maximum muscle. And in between, you can vary the degree of each by making simple tweaks to your diet.

The idea here isn't to give you a complicated set of choices. These options allow you to tweak the plan to work best not only for your goals but also for your lifestyle. For example, if you have 25 pounds to lose, you'll get the fastest results with Plan A, which is a low-carbohydrate diet. But if you want more flexibility in your diet, you might choose Plan C. This plan lets you load up on carbs 1 day a week and provides the added benefit of more muscle growth. Adapt the TNT Diet to your goals and lifestyle—not the other way around. Here's an overview of Plans A through E; we'll explore the details of each further in Chapter 3.

TARGETED NUTRITION TACTICS	PLAN A	PLAN B	PLAN C	PLAN D	PLAN E
The Fat-Burning Time Zone (low-carbohydrate)	7 days	7 days	6 days	6 days	5 days
The Reloading Time Zone (high-carbohydrate)	0 days	0 days	1 day	1 day	2 days
The Muscle-Building Time Zone (workout nutrition)	Protein only	Protein + carbs	Protein only	Protein + carbs	Protein + carbs

THE FINAL TACTIC

Most people realize that you can't build a beach body without exercise. But what seems lost on many is that weight training is the key, not aerobic exercise. That's because lifting weights not only burns as many calories as, say, a moderate-intensity run, it also elevates your metabolism for almost 2 days afterward. Lifting is also highly effective at reducing glycogen levels, and, of course, stimulates muscle growth. We'll cover the specific workout details more fully in Chapters 10 and 11, but for now, just know that weight training is the most efficient and effective form of exercise you can do. Although the workout we've created appears simple, it's based on the culmination of decades of muscle research, the laws of human physiology, and hundreds of interviews with the world's top strength coaches and trainers.

"I had to keep tightening my belt."

Name: **Lucas Hutchinson**
Age: **25**
Height: **6 feet 4 inches**
Weight before: **250**
Weight after: **243**

IF YOU WERE TO JUDGE LUCAS HUTCHINSON'S RESULTS by the numbers on the scale, you wouldn't be too impressed. After all, in 12 weeks on the TNT Diet, he lost only 7 pounds of body weight.

But remember, it's body *composition* that matters. And by that standard, Lucas made one of the most dramatic transformations we've seen in any of our studies. That's because he lost 19 pounds of fat, while packing on 12 pounds of muscle.

In fact, his results were so amazing that we double- and triple-checked the readings to be sure they were correct. Not that we should have been that surprised: The change in his body was obvious. And not just to us: "In the first month, I noticed that my pants were fitting a little looser. As the study progressed, I had to keep tightening my belt, and it felt great every time I did it."

Lucas added more muscle—a pound a week—than anyone in our studies to date. And although we can't tell you exactly why—hey, everyone responds a little differently—we do know that he made it a point to enjoy the meal plan. "The best part of the diet by far is the fat. I was able to use as much as I wanted, and it always made my meals taste better," says Lucas. There's an important lesson here: By not fearing fat, and eating all the calories that he desired, he allowed the TNT Diet to work its magic—diverting nutrients away from the fat depots that surrounded his belly, and toward the muscles of his chest, back, and legs.

What about his health? Judge for yourself. Lucas's total cholesterol fell 17 percent and his triglycerides dropped an astounding 58 percent. On top of it all, there was another benefit: "I slept better and had more energy when I woke up," he says.

CHAPTER 3

YOUR BODY, YOUR PLAN

To be honest, we aren't all that fond of regimented eating plans. Mainly because they're, well, regimented. This tends to lead to the unfortunate mindset that if you deviate from the plan a little, then you've abandoned it altogether—a thought pattern we hope you never develop.

But we also realize that a clear plan can be a valuable learning tool. By following detailed guidelines, you'll quickly begin to better comprehend the underlying principles that inspired them. More importantly, you'll be able to accurately judge how your body responds to a very specific manner of eating. That way, you can make an objective assessment of how well an eating plan works for you. Got that? Not how well it works for your buddy, your wife, or 20 people who took part in a scientific study. But how well it works for *you*. And isn't that the whole point?

All of which is why we've created the five TNT plans that follow. We've set some ground rules for each, to help you decide which one to adopt, and to ensure that you have the greatest success possible. The idea is that you'll choose your plan based not only on your body composition goals—faster fat loss? more muscle?—but also on how much fat you have to lose.

However, we want everyone to start out by following the guidelines of TNT Plan A for the first 4 weeks. The reason: To experience all the benefits from the other plans we offer, your body must first learn to use fat as its primary source of energy. Think of this as lighting the TNT Diet fuse. Typically, your body will adapt almost completely within a week or two, and the rest of the changes will occur within another 2 weeks. So for the first 4 weeks, you'll follow TNT Plan A, regardless of your goals. After that, you can stay on Plan A, or switch to any of the other four plans you want based on your goals. But no matter what, you'll start to see the fat-blasting benefits of the TNT Diet right from the start.

BEFORE YOU LIGHT THE FUSE

Fair warning: The first week or two on Plan A may be a little difficult. Your body has to adapt to burning fat as its main energy source. For most people, this is a major change because they're accustomed—some would even say addicted—to using carbohydrates to fuel their body.

You may be irritable, cranky, and even tired for a few days. But as you grow accustomed to this new diet, you'll return to your lovable self quickly. Within a couple of weeks, guys following Plan A almost always report having higher and more consistent energy levels than they did before they started the program. In fact, many TNT veterans claim that they need less sleep when eating this way. If the change from your normal diet is a particularly drastic one, you may also experience a bit of gastrointestinal distress, such as diarrhea. However, within a few days, we can assure you that your plumbing will be working normally again. And as long as you stick to the guidelines of Plan A, any cravings for carbs will soon disappear as well. You'll actually be more in tune with your body's true hunger signals, as opposed to being a slave to the cravings that are triggered by the typical high-carb "sugar rush," followed by the inevitable "sugar crash." On Plan A, you'll be immune to these highs and lows while you're humming along in your new fat-burning mode.

It's important to remember that Plan A is absolutely a low-carbohydrate, *high-fat* diet. We emphasize this point because a common mistake people make during Plan A is that they try to limit both carbs and fat. This often makes the diet unpleasant and hard to follow. It also makes it difficult for you to consume enough calories to properly fuel your body. The bottom line: Don't be afraid of fat! Ideally, you'll be eating anywhere from 60 to 70 percent of your calories from fat. Of course, you won't need to calculate this

---

Give Yourself a Checkup

One way to monitor your progress is to invest in a CardioChek Portable Blood Test System. This device allows you to measure total cholesterol, HDL cholesterol, triglycerides, glucose, and even ketones with just a finger prick and in the comfort and convenience of your home.

It's no substitute for a trip to your doctor, but it does allow you to check markers of heart disease risk on a regular basis. CardioChek is available at Wal-Mart ($99 when we went to press), but you can also visit the CardioChek Web site (www.cardiochek.com) for more information and additional retailers.

out, but it's a pretty good bet that if you aren't enjoying the diet, you aren't eating enough fat. Again, our research shows that eating a low-carb, high-fat diet actually reduces your risk for heart disease, despite what you've been told—so have a little faith.

Finally, we highly recommend that you get a checkup with full blood work before you start this plan. Why? Because it's the best way to know how well the diet is benefiting your health. We've provided you with examples of what happens to people normally, but the only way to really know is to see for yourself. And after all, why would you leave your health to chance? Tell your doctor that you're following a new diet and you want to gauge its effect on your cardiovascular health. Then have him or her, at the very least, measure the following: triglycerides, HDL cholesterol, LDL cholesterol, fasting glucose, fasting insulin, and blood pressure. Before you leave, schedule a follow-up appointment for 4 weeks later, in which you'll have your blood work done again. This will provide a snapshot of the impact your plan is having on your health. (For an idea of what to expect, see Chapter 12.)

PICK YOUR PLAN

TNT PLAN A

*Choose this plan if **any** of these statements apply to you:*

- You're just starting the program.
- You have more than 20 pounds of fat to lose.
- You want to drop more than 4 inches from your waist.
- You want to lose fat at the highest rate possible.
- You have metabolic syndrome or prediabetes.

What to do: Implement each Time Zone as directed and follow the guidelines for each, provided in Part II.

- The Fat-Burning Time Zone: Every day of the week, except 1 hour before your workout and 1 hour after your workout.
- The Reloading Time Zone: Not implemented.
- The Muscle-Building Time Zone: Between 1 hour before each workout until 1 hour after, adhere to the Protein Only option. (For complete instructions, see Chapter 7.)

TNT PLAN B

*Choose this plan if **all** of these statements apply to you:*

- You've already completed 4 weeks on TNT Plan A.
- You have less than 20 pounds of fat to lose.
- You want to drop less than 4 inches from your waist.
- You want to boost the impact of your workout on muscle growth but emphasize fat burning at all other times.

What to do: Implement each Time Zone as directed and follow the guidelines for each, provided in Part II.

- The Fat-Burning Time Zone: Every day of the week, except 1 hour before your workout and 1 hour after your workout.
- The Reloading Time Zone: Not implemented.
- The Muscle-Building Time Zone: Between 1 hour before each workout until 1 hour after, adhere to the Protein + Carbohydrates option. (For complete instructions, see Chapter 7.)

TNT PLAN C

*Choose this plan if **all** of these statements apply to you:*

- You've already completed 4 weeks on TNT Plan A.
- You have less than 20 pounds of fat to lose.
- You want to drop less than 4 inches from your waist.
- You want to burn fat at the highest rate possible 6 days a week but would like a day in which you can have lots of carbohydrates, without having to worry about undoing your efforts or stalling your progress.

What to do: Implement each Time Zone as directed and follow the guidelines for each, provided in Part II.

- The Fat-Burning Time Zone: Sunday through Friday, except 1 hour before your workout and 1 hour after your workout.
- The Reloading Time Zone: All day Saturday.
- The Muscle-Building Time Zone: Between 1 hour before each workout until 1 hour after, adhere to the Protein Only option. (For complete instructions, see Chapter 7.)

TNT PLAN D

*Choose this plan if **all** of these statements apply to you:*

- You've already completed 4 weeks on TNT Plan A.
- You have less than 10 pounds of fat to lose.
- You want to drop less than 3 inches from your waist.
- You want to ramp up muscle growth, while still burning fat most of the time.

What to do: Implement each Time Zone as directed and follow the guidelines for each, provided in Part II.

- The Fat-Burning Time Zone: Monday through Saturday, except 1 hour before your workout and 1 hour after your workout.
- The Reloading Time Zone: All day Sunday.
- The Muscle-Building Time Zone: Between 1 hour before each workout until 1 hour after, adhere to the Protein + Carbohydrates option. (For complete instructions, see Chapter 7.)

TNT PLAN E

*Choose this plan if **all** of these statements apply to you:*

- You've already completed 4 weeks on TNT Plan A.
- You have less than 5 pounds of fat to lose.
- You want to drop less than 2 inches from your waist.
- You want to maximize muscle growth, without gaining fat.

What to do: Implement each Time Zone as directed and follow the guidelines for each, provided in Part II.

- The Fat-Burning Time Zone: From Sunday at 10 a.m. through Friday at 6 p.m., except 1 hour before your workout and 1 hour after your workout.
- The Reloading Time Zone: Friday 6 p.m. through Sunday 10 a.m.
- The Muscle-Building Time Zone: Between 1 hour before each workout until 1 hour after, adhere to the Protein + Carbohydrates option. (For complete instructions, see Chapter 7.)

ONCE THE FUSE IS LIT

Soon after you light the TNT fuse, you can expect to see and feel rapid changes in your physique. The key, of course, is sticking with the plan for a full 12 weeks. We believe the secret to this is making a point to embrace the foods that you can eat in each Time Zone, particularly the Fat-Burning Zone. Over and over, we've seen that the guys who experience the best results on this plan are the ones who focus on what they can eat, instead of on what they can't eat. They adopt the mindset that food is to be enjoyed, and take advantage of the fact that the TNT Diet doesn't force you to limit your food intake or count calories. This approach ensures that you never feel like you're dieting. Which means you'll simply be eating a lot of the foods that you love. And who couldn't stick with a diet like that?

For help with all your TNT questions, visit www.MensHealth.com/TNT. You'll find a complete FAQ section, an interactive discussion forum, and an online community created specifically for TNT dieters.

PART II: WHAT TO EAT WHEN

CHAPTER 4

THE TNT DIET QUICK-START GUIDE

What's standing between you and the body you want? With the TNT Diet, the answer is nothing. Whether you want to melt your midsection and uncover your abs, or lay down slabs of new muscle, the TNT Diet has a plan for you. After reading the overview of the diet in Chapter 3, you know that 4 weeks on Plan A is the place to start. Once you've completed this introductory phase, you'll need to decide which of our five plans best suits your goals. Follow the rules provided in this chapter for each Time Zone, according to the guidelines of the plan you chose. Keep in mind, this is just a snapshot of each Time Zone. You'll find the complete details for each—and the answers to all your questions—in the chapters that follow. As you begin the diet portion of TNT, you'll also want to start the exercise plan, which begins on page 147. Remember, the workout program is crucial for harnessing the full power of TNT.

THE FAT-BURNING TIME ZONE

THE NUTRITION TACTICS

1. Eat any combination of the Fat-Burning Time Zone foods, until you feel satisfied, but not stuffed.

2. Try to consume high-quality protein at every meal.

3. Don't fear fat.

4. Indulge on vegetables.

5. Avoid sugar and starch.

THE FAT-BURNING TIME ZONE FOODS

HIGH-QUALITY PROTEIN	LOW-STARCH VEGETABLES*		NATURAL FATS
Beef	Artichokes	Mushrooms	Avocados
Cheese	Asparagus	Onions	Butter
Eggs	Broccoli	Peppers	Coconut
Fish	Brussels sprouts	Spinach	Cream
Pork	Cauliflower	Tomatoes	Nuts and seeds†
Poultry	Celery	Turnips	Olives, olive oil, and canola oil
Whey and casein protein	Cucumbers	Zucchini	Sour cream

*These are just a few common examples of low-starch vegetables; the full list (page 44) includes almost all vegetables except potatoes, carrots, and corn.

†Limit nuts and seeds to two servings a day.

THE RELOADING TIME ZONE

THE NUTRITION TACTICS

1. Eat any combination of the Reloading Time Zone foods until you feel satisfied, but not stuffed.

2. Try to eat high-quality protein at every meal and every 3 hours.

THE RELOADING TIME ZONE FOODS

HIGH-QUALITY PROTEIN	FRUITS AND VEGETABLES*		NUTRIENT-DENSE CARBOHYDRATES
Beef	Asparagus	Apples	Beans
Cheese	Broccoli	Bananas	Bread
Eggs and egg whites	Carrots	Berries	Cereal
Fish	Corn	Grapes	Flour
Kefir	Onions	Melon	Oats
Milk	Peppers	Oranges	Pasta
Pork	Potatoes	Peaches	Quinoa
Poultry	Spinach	Pears	Rice
Yogurt	Tomatoes	Pineapple	Tortillas

*These are just a few common examples of fruits and vegetables; just about any type of produce imaginable is acceptable.

3. Consume nutrient-dense carbohydrates or fruit at each meal.

4. Go easy on extra fats, such as nuts, seeds, and butter.

5. Avoid added sugar and refined grains, such as white bread; opt for 100 percent whole grain products instead.

THE MUSCLE-BUILDING TIME ZONE

THE NUTRITION TACTICS: PROTEIN ONLY

(TNT Plans A and C)

Prepare a protein shake (made with water) that provides at least 40 grams of whey and/or casein protein. When choosing a product, look for one that contains only small amounts of carbs and fat.

- Drink half of the beverage 30 to 45 minutes before your workout; drink the other half immediately after your workout.

- Eat a Fat-Burning Time Zone meal or snack that contains high-quality protein within 30 minutes to 1 hour after your training session. (Your snack could be another 20- to 40-gram protein shake.)

- For more options, refer to the complete Muscle-Building Time Zone guidelines in Chapter 7.

THE NUTRITION TACTICS: PROTEIN + CARBOHYDRATES

(TNT Plans B, D, and E)

Prepare a protein shake (made with water or milk) that provides at least 40 grams of whey and/or casein protein and 40 to 80 grams of carbohydrates. When choosing a product, look for one that contains little or no fat. As a good alternative, opt for a 16-ounce carton of low-fat chocolate milk or low-fat, fruit-flavored kefir.

- Drink half of the beverage 30 minutes before your workout; drink the other half immediately after your workout.

- Eat a Fat-Burning Time Zone meal or snack that contains high-quality protein within 30 minutes to 1 hour after your training session. (Keep in mind, your Fat-Burning Time Zone snack could be another 20- to 40-gram protein shake, made without the carbs.)

THE DRINK LIST

THE NUTRITION TACTICS

With the exception of alcohol, consume as much of these beverages as you want. For water, try to drink 8 to 12 ounces for every 2 hours that you're awake.

TNT-Approved Beverages

Water

Coffee

Any type of unsweetened tea

No-calorie beverages

Alcohol: up to two drinks per day

CHAPTER 5

THE FAT-BURNING TIME ZONE

No matter which TNT plan you've chosen, the foods in the Fat-Burning Time Zone will form the foundation of your diet. That's because they're low in carbohydrates, which ensures that they won't raise your levels of insulin or glycogen. Keeping high amounts of carbs out of your diet lets your body burn fat at its highest potential, while protecting metabolism-boosting muscle. The Fat-Burning Time Zone diet also helps to stabilize your blood sugar and reduce your body's internal production of saturated fat. Both of these results are extremely effective for decreasing your risk for heart disease. Even better: The guidelines in the Fat-Burning Time Zone are simple; just follow the five nutrition tactics below.

THE NUTRITION TACTICS

1. Choose liberally from the Fat-Burning Time Zone foods. Feel free to eat any combination of these foods—along with the Fat-Burning Time Zone–approved condiments and beverages—until you feel satisfied, but not stuffed. These "restrictions" sound too easy to work, but study after study has shown that eating this way promises more dramatic fat loss than any other approach—and without the need to count calories.

2. Try to consume high-quality protein at every meal. Eating protein ensures that your body always has the raw material available to build and maintain your muscle, even while you lose fat. Protein also helps to keep your metabolism stoked. That's because your body uses more calories to digest and process protein than both carbohydrates and fat combined.

3. Don't fear fat. Fat is a crucial factor in helping you control the total number of calories your body craves. That's because fat is very effective at helping you feel satisfied. Remember, your body is designed to burn fat. And *you* control the fat-burning trigger by eating foods—specifically, the Fat-Burning Time Zone foods—that keep your insulin and glycogen levels low.

4. Indulge on vegetables. When our friend and colleague, Richard Feinman, PhD, professor of biochemistry at SUNY Downstate Medical Center in New York City, polled more than 2,000 low-carbohydrate dieters, he found that, on average, dieters who were most successful consumed at least four servings of low-starch vegetables a day. Low-starch vegetables include almost any vegetable other than potatoes, carrots, and corn.

5. Avoid sugar and starch. The list of foods to avoid includes bread, pasta, potatoes, beans, rice, fruit, milk, candy, regular soda, and baked goods—as well as any other foods that contain grains, flour, or sugar. The reason? These are the foods that either raise blood sugar and insulin levels or replenish glycogen—all of which inhibit your body's ability to burn fat for energy. You might be surprised to see fruit and milk on this list, but it's not because either are unhealthy—they simply provide too many glycogen-replenishing carbs, in the form of natural sugars.

THE FAT-BURNING TIME ZONE FOODS

HIGH-QUALITY PROTEIN	LOW-STARCH VEGETABLES*		NATURAL FATS
Beef	Artichokes	Mushrooms	Avocados
Cheese	Asparagus	Onions	Butter
Eggs	Broccoli	Peppers	Coconut
Fish	Brussels sprouts	Spinach	Cream
Pork	Cauliflower	Tomatoes	Nuts and seeds[†]
Poultry	Celery	Turnips	Olives, olive oil, and canola oil
Whey and casein protein	Cucumbers	Zucchini	Sour cream

*These are just a few common examples of low-starch vegetables; the full list (page 44) includes almost all vegetables except potatoes, carrots, and corn.

[†]Limit nuts and seeds to two servings a day.

Sugar by Any Other Name . . .

Scanning a product's ingredient list to see if it has sugar is smart—but you may need to expand your vocabulary. Here are 20 aliases that the sweet stuff goes by—none of which include the word *sugar*.

Barley malt	High-fructose corn syrup
Brown rice syrup	Honey
Corn syrup	Lactose
Dextrose	Maltodextrin
Evaporated cane juice invert syrup	Maple syrup
Fructose	Molasses
Fruit juice	Organic cane juice
Galactose	Sorghum
Glucose	Sucrose
Granular fruit grape juice concentrate	Turbinado

HIGH-QUALITY PROTEIN

BEEF

Most people consider turkey, chicken, and fish healthy, yet think they should avoid red meat—or only choose very lean cuts—since they've always been told that it's high in saturated fat. But there are two problems with that thinking.

The first problem is that almost half of the fat in beef is a *monounsaturated* fat called *oleic acid*—the same heart-healthy fat that's found in olive oil. Second, most of the saturated fat in beef actually decrease*s* your heart disease risk—either by lowering LDL (bad) cholesterol, or by reducing your ratio of total cholesterol to HDL (good) cholesterol. (See Chapter 13 for the science on saturated fat and your health.) And besides being one of the most available sources of high-quality protein, beef also provides many important nutrients such as iron, zinc, and B vitamins. So the idea that beef is bad for you couldn't be further from the truth.

POULTRY

We probably don't have to sell you on the virtues of chicken and turkey. After all, nearly all experts agree that these foods are healthy sources of high-quality protein. But unlike most nutritionists, we also say go ahead and eat both the dark meat and the skin. Because both are composed of animal fat, their fat composition is very similar to that of beef. Meaning, neither raises your risk for heart disease. Remember, eating more fat—not less—is key in helping you reduce your calorie intake without feeling deprived.

FISH

Any type of fish is a good source of high-quality protein, but those that inhabit cold water are even better choices. Research shows that regular consumption of cold-water fish—such as salmon, mackerel, halibut, and sardines—lowers the risk of heart disease, stroke, asthma, colon cancer, kidney cancer, and Alzheimer's. Why? Scientists believe it's because they're rich in a type of fat known as *omega-3 fatty acids.* Specifically, these beneficial omega-3s are called *eicosapentaenoic acid* and *docosahexaenoic acid,* or EPA and DHA, respectively. For most of the health benefits, you should consume enough fatty fish each week to provide at least 3,000 milligrams of EPA and DHA combined. Use the chart below to guide your selections. (Hate fish? Try the fish oil supplement recommended on page 56.)

SOURCE	EPA AND DHA PER 3½-OUNCE SERVING
Salmon	2,200 mg
Mackerel	1,200 mg
Sardines	1,000 mg
Trout	1,000 mg
Mussels	800 mg
Sea bass	800 mg
White tuna (canned in water)	800 mg
Calamari	600 mg
Flounder	500 mg
Halibut	500 mg
Lox	500 mg
Crab	400 mg

PORK

It's true: Pork really is the other white meat. Ounce for ounce, pork tenderloin has less fat than chicken breast. And food scientists are finding ways to make it leaner and leaner every year. Of course, the downside to this is that fat is what makes pork taste so good—which explains why ham and bacon are far more popular than leaner cuts. (As Emeril Lagasse says, "Pork fat rules.") But remember, there's no reason to fear fat—especially when you follow the tenets of the TNT Diet.

Not everyone has a taste for bacon, pancetta, and ham. But you can make your choice based simply on what you love without worrying about the fat in these foods. When you follow the TNT Diet, your health and body composition results will be every bit as impressive with these foods as without—so why deny your taste buds? One caveat: Bacon and other cured meats often contain sodium and other preservatives, such as nitrates, that may raise blood pressure, or increase your risk for cancer. To limit your risk, choose fresh meats or packaged products that contain no preservatives—typically labeled "all-natural"—whenever possible. Our favorite: Al Fresco chicken sausages; find a local retailer at www.alfrescoallnatural.com.

EGGS

Whole eggs contain more essential vitamins and minerals per calorie than virtually any other food. They're also one of the best sources of choline, a substance your body requires to break down fat for energy. In addition, eggs provide lutein and zeaxanthin, antioxidants that help prevent macular degeneration and cataracts. They may even be the perfect diet food: Saint Louis University scientists found that people who have eggs as part of their breakfast eat fewer calories the rest of the day than those who ate bagels instead. Even though both breakfasts contained the same number of calories, the egg eaters consumed 264 fewer calories for the entire day.

However, you've probably been told at one time or another to avoid eggs because they're high in cholesterol and fat. This is the same thinking that led to low-fat diets—and a mindset that has probably made us a lot fatter over the past decade. It's simply a leftover recommendation from the low-fat legacy that was never forgotten. In a recent review of dozens of scientific studies, Wake Forest University researchers found no connection between egg consumption and heart disease. Which may be why, as the scientists point out in their paper, even the American Heart Association's guidelines no longer include the recommendation to limit your intake of eggs.

CHEESE

There are three main reasons that cheese—believe it or not—is considered a great diet food.

1. It's packed with protein and fat, which keep you full.

2. Most cheeses have almost no carbohydrates, which means they don't raise your insulin levels or refill your glycogen tank.

3. Cheese is versatile and convenient. You can eat it right out of a single-serving package—making it a great snack—or use as a dip or to add more flavor to almost any dish.

You can choose from any type of hard cheese, or nonflavored cream cheese. However, in the Fat-Burning Time Zone, you'll want to avoid cottage and ricotta cheese, since they contain a significant amount of carbohydrates. The same goes for flavored cream cheeses—think: strawberry—and processed cheese spreads. An easy way to make the determination: If the label shows that the cheese contains 2 grams or more of carbohydrates per serving (1 ounce or 1 slice), choose a different kind. Otherwise, it's an excellent choice.

TNT-APPROVED CHEESES*

American	Cream cheese, plain	Gouda	Mozzarella
Blue	Edam	Halloumi	Muenster
Brie	Feta	Havarti	Parmesan
Brick	Fontina	Jarlsberg	Provolone
Camembert	Goat	Mascarpone	Romano
Cheddar	Gorgonzola	Monterey Jack	Swiss

*There are hundreds of different types of cheeses that you can eat; these are just a few examples. You'll be able to determine if a product fits the Fat-Burning Time Zone by checking the label.

WHEY AND CASEIN PROTEIN

Because whey and casein protein supplements are popular among the body-building crowd, you might assume that these products are only for "hard-core" lifters. But the truth is, they're simply a convenient way to increase your intake of high-quality protein. A quick primer: Whey and casein are the primary proteins found in milk. In fact, about 20 percent of the protein in milk is whey, and the other 80 percent is casein. Any time you drink a glass of milk, you're consuming both whey and casein. Over the last few years, scientists have learned how to separate these proteins from milk and then create powders that can be used to supplement your diet. Products

Whey Versus Casein

Although both proteins are high quality—meaning they contain all of the essential amino acids needed to build muscle—they're processed differently by your body. Whey is known as a "fast protein," meaning it's quickly broken down into amino acids and absorbed into your bloodstream. This allows the amino acids to be delivered to your muscles for immediate use. For this reason, it's a very good protein to consume after your workout, when your body's ability to build and repair muscle is at its highest. Casein, on the other hand, is digested more slowly. So it's ideal for providing your body with a steady supply of smaller amounts of protein for a longer period of time. As a result, it's a great choice for before you go to bed. For most purposes, both proteins will provide a similar overall benefit. However, if you're interested in optimizing your protein intake, you might consider a whey-casein blend, which gives you the benefits of both proteins. Another choice: a protein made with "milk protein isolates," which, because they're milk protein, contain both whey and casein.

made from either protein are both excellent sources of high-quality protein. Another benefit: Consumption of whey protein has been shown to enhance immune function and to be beneficial in treating cancer, heart disease, and osteoporosis. For a list of our favorite protein supplements, see Chapter 7. (Choose those that contain only protein, and little or no carbohydrates.)

LOW-STARCH VEGETABLES

We could give the nutritional merits of each vegetable listed on page 44, but we thought we'd save ourselves the work, and you the time. After all, do you really need to be convinced that vegetables are good for you? They are, of course. Harvard University researchers found that for every additional serving increase in daily vegetable intake, your risk of heart disease decreases 4 percent. And eating vegetables has also been shown to lower your risk of stroke, cancer, and diabetes.

When shopping, you can choose from just about any form of vegetable, including fresh, frozen, or canned. And you can serve your vegetables raw, or cooked, by steaming, grilling, sautéing, boiling, or roasting.

Again, the key is simply to avoid vegetables that are starchy, which, for the most part, means potatoes in any of its various forms—mashed, fried, baked, and sweet. Also included in that list, though, are carrots, corn, and parsnips. We make a point to separate these from potatoes for a reason: You're not likely to eat an abundance of these vegetables, and one serving of any of them has significantly lower amounts of carbohydrates and calories than one serving of potato. So if the steamed vegetables you order happen to have a few carrots mixed in with the broccoli, don't feel like you have to let them go to waste. The main concern is that you don't eat them regularly or in large quantities when you're in the Fat-Burning Time Zone.

Besides combining your vegetables with natural fats, such as butter, you can use any of the Fat-Burning Time Zone–approved herbs and spices to add flavor and variety.

Just for reference, consider one serving of vegetables to be either 1 cup raw (the size of a baseball) or ½ cup cooked (half the size of a baseball). Although it's not necessary to know this to lose fat, gauging your intake may actually help you pay attention to eating enough. Remember, the most successful dieters eat, on average, four servings of vegetables a day.

THE FAT-BURNING TIME ZONE-APPROVED LOW-STARCH VEGETABLES

Alfalfa sprouts	Cauliflower	Mushrooms	Spaghetti squash
Artichokes	Celery	Okra	Spinach
Arugula	Cucumber	Onions	Summer squash
Asparagus	Eggplant	Peppers (any color)	Tomatoes
Bean sprouts	Endive	Radishes	Turnips
Bok choy	Green beans	Sauerkraut	Watercress
Broccoli	Kale	Scallions	Zucchini
Brussels sprouts	Lettuce (any type)	Snow peas	

Why You Should Mix It Up

Colorado State University scientists discovered that people who consume the widest array of vegetables experience more health benefits than those who eat just as much but choose from a smaller assortment of produce. Why? The protective mojo of plant foods comes from antioxidants called *phytochemicals,* compounds that guard cells against damaging oxidation. However, these phytochemicals vary from one botanical family to another. So the greater the variety of vegetables you eat, the more types of healthy phytochemicals you consume.

NATURAL FATS

AVOCADOS

Technically, an avocado is a fruit. But because they're so rich in natural fats, we include them in this category. The bonus: They're also loaded with disease-fighting antioxidants. However, avocados do contain a significant amount of carbohydrates, so don't eat more than half an avocado on any given day.

BUTTER

If this delicious dairy product were the star of a sitcom, the show would probably be called *Everybody Hates Butter*. The reason, of course, is that it contains a significant amount of saturated fat. But again, it's animal fat, like the kind in beef, bacon, and chicken skin. This is a natural fat that men and women have eaten for thousands of years—yet heart disease didn't appear until the 20th century. The uptick in heart disease coincides not with an increase in saturated fat intake, but with that of more sugar and refined grains in our daily diets. And consider this: Fat, like that in butter, is *necessary* in order to help your body absorb many of the healthy nutrients found in vegetables. For instance, without fat, your body can't absorb carotenoids—powerful disease-fighting antioxidants found in colorful vegetables—or fat-soluble vitamins, such as vitamins A, D, E, and K. So go ahead, eat butter, and do it without guilt when you're in the Fat-Burning Time Zone.

COCONUT

Ounce for ounce, coconut contains even more saturated fat than butter does. As a result, health experts have warned that it will clog your arteries. But even though coconut is packed with saturated fat, it too appears to have a beneficial effect on heart-disease risk factors. One reason: More than 50 percent of its saturated-fat content is lauric acid. A recent analysis of 60 studies published in the *American Journal of Clinical Nutrition* reports that even though lauric acid raises LDL (bad) cholesterol, it boosts HDL (good) cholesterol even more. Overall, this means it decreases your risk of cardiovascular disease. The rest of the saturated fat in a coconut is believed to have little or no effect on cholesterol levels. We think coconut is highly underrated—if you like the taste, try it as a snack, eating the *unsweetened,* shredded kind straight from the bag. (You'll probably have to search the health food section of your grocery store to find it.)

NUTS

It's time to leave the trail mix and rice cakes where they belong: the 1980s. Here in the 21st century, we know that nuts and seeds are far healthier snack foods. Many people mistakenly avoid nuts because of their high fat content, which ranges from about 70 to 80 percent of their total calories. This is possibly one of the best examples of how misinformation has really done a disservice to the American public (and the American plate). Study after study in prestigious journals such as the *Journal of the American Medical Association* show that an increased consumption of nuts can have a preventive effect on a number of diseases and health conditions, including obesity, heart disease, insulin resistance, and diabetes. And increased nut consumption doesn't lead to weight gain. The bonus is that nuts and seeds also have plenty of fiber and protein, which along with the fat, keep you full longer than high-carb snacks—without boosting your insulin levels.

> One serving of nuts or seeds is equal to a small handful, or the size of a large egg; one serving of nut butter is about the same size as a golf ball.

Two caveats:

1. Limit your daily intake to two to three servings of nuts and seeds. Why? One serving—about 1 ounce—contains 6 to 8 grams of carbohydrates. Eat too many, and this can start to add up. These extra carbs will

The Best Brand of Peanut Butter

Not only do most commercial brands of peanut butter contain added sugar, many are sweetened with "icing sugar"—the same finely ground sugar used to decorate cupcakes. In fact, each tablespoon of regular Skippy peanut butter contains a half teaspoon of the sweet stuff. And reduced-fat versions are even worse. That's because manufacturers simply replace some of the healthy fat with even more icing sugar. They might as well print "stick a birthday candle in me" right on the label.

Trouble is, many people don't like natural peanut butter because the oil separates from the spread during storage, requiring you to remix it before eating. (That's assuming you don't spill the oil all over yourself when you open the jar.) One trick: Store your all-natural peanut butter in the refrigerator, which slows the separation process. Our favorite brand: Crazy Richard's Natural Chunky Peanut Butter. It contains no added sugar or trans fats, and we've found that it's slower to separate than other all-natural brands.

not only help replenish glycogen levels, but they also impair the ability of the TNT Diet to regulate your total calorie intake.

2. Avoid nuts and seeds with added sugar. These include nuts that are honey-roasted, candy-coated, and barbecued. The bottom line: Choose from those that are raw, dry-roasted, oil-roasted, blanched, chopped, slivered, shelled, salted, or unsalted. Also, buy natural nut butters—such as peanut butter and almond butter—over commercial brands that contain added sugar.

THE FAT-BURNING TIME ZONE-APPROVED NUTS AND SEEDS

Almonds	Peanut butter
Almond butter	Pecans
Brazil nuts	Pine nuts
Cashews	Pistachios
Hazelnuts	Pumpkin seeds
Macadamia nuts	Sesame seeds
Mixed nuts	Sunflower seeds
Peanuts	Walnuts

OLIVES, OLIVE OIL, AND CANOLA OIL

The fat contained in olives, whether it's from the fruit itself, or the oil derived from it, is primarily monounsaturated fat. The same is true for canola oil. Monounsaturated fat is universally considered healthy. Research shows that increasing your consumption of this healthy fat lowers your risk for heart disease. So, again, you can liberally include these foods in your diet. We also suggest that as a general rule, you choose olive and canola oils over other types of vegetable oils, such as corn and soybean. That's because corn and soybean oils are extremely high in omega-6 fatty acids. These aren't bad when they're balanced with plenty of omega-3 fatty acids—like the kind found in fish—but that often isn't the case in the typical American diet. For instance, corn oil has 60 times more omega-6s than omega-3s. And studies suggest that a high intake of omega-6 fats relative to omega-3 fats increases inflammation, which boosts your risk of cancer, arthritis, and obesity. Our belief, one that is supported by research, is that you're already consuming too many omega-6 fats. So by emphasizing olive and canola oils over other veg-etable oils, you'll automatically reduce your intake, and create a healthier balance of omega-6 to omega-3 fats.

SOUR CREAM

For years, you've been told to avoid sour cream or to eat the light version. That's because 90 percent of its calories are derived from fat, at least half of which is saturated. Sure, the percentage of fat is high, but the total amount isn't. Consider that a serving of sour cream is 2 tablespoons. That provides just 52 calories—half the amount that's in a single tablespoon of mayon-naise—and less saturated fat than you'd get from drinking a 12-ounce glass of 2% reduced-fat milk. More importantly, sour cream is a close relative of butter, which means you're eating natural animal fat, not dangerous trans fat. And besides, full-fat sour cream tastes far better than the light or fat-free products, which also have added carbohydrates.

THE FAT-BURNING TIME ZONE-APPROVED CONDIMENTS, SPICES, AND HERBS

These foods are your secret weapon because they allow you to add a variety of flavors to any meal. Below, we've listed the most common condiments,

Aioli	Fennel seed	Pesto
Balsamic vinegar	Fish sauce	Rice vinegar
Basil	Garlic	Rosemary
Capers	Ginger	Saffron
Caraway seeds	Horseradish	Sage
Cayenne	Mayonnaise	Salt
Chili powder	Mint	Soy sauce
Chives	Mustard	Tabasco sauce
Cilantro	Oregano	Thyme
Cinnamon	Paprika	Turmeric
Cumin	Parsley	Vinegar
Dill	Pepper	Worcestershire sauce

spices, and herbs that are compatible with the Fat-Burning Time Zone. For the most part, the list includes just about everything but ketchup and barbecue sauce. (If you're a ketchup lover, you can use a low-carb ketchup, such as the one Heinz makes.) However, we may have missed a few that you enjoy. If it's an herb or a spice, consider it acceptable regardless. If it's a condiment, check the label: You'll want to avoid products that contain more than 2 grams of carbohydrates per serving. As for salad dressings and marinades, the same rules apply, although it's sometimes hard to find such products beyond, say, blue cheese, ranch, and Italian dressings.

We highly recommend Drew's All-Natural dressings and marinades (available at www.chefdrew.com), which come in a variety of flavors, but contain little or no added sugars.

THE FAT-BURNING TIME ZONE MENU

By simply sticking to the Fat-Burning Time Zone foods, you can't mess up this portion of the diet. However, we've created a short list of foods below to show you the different types of meals you can have for breakfast, lunch, and dinner, as well as snack options that are available. Keep in mind, these are just suggestions, and far from an all-inclusive menu or rigid meal plan. By all means be creative—for instance, feel free to have dinner for breakfast, or breakfast for dinner; it's irrelevant when it comes to your results. What does matter is that you limit your choices to the Fat-Burning Time Zone foods, and that you eat when hungry and until full.

BREAKFAST

Scrambled eggs

Poached eggs

Omelet

- Denver
- Greek
- Ham and cheese
- Western
- Any other combination of meats, vegetables, and cheeses

Fried eggs

Dining Out without Falling Off

If you've dieted before, you know how hard it can be to maintain your plan while eating lunch or dinner at a restaurant. But the beauty of the TNT Diet is that you won't feel restricted—not the way you do on other plans. That's because this diet isn't about limiting choices; it's about making the *right* choices. For instance, you can enjoy the finest dishes at your favorite five-star steak restaurant; they just have to be the right dishes. It's a lot easier than you might imagine. Just follow these three simple rules any time you eat out, whether it's the neighborhood grill, an upscale eatery, or even a fast-food restaurant.

1. Substitute fresh vegetables for potatoes, pasta, and rice.

This very simple step is also the one that will have the greatest impact. It will dramatically reduce the total number of calories you eat while also making you feel more satisfied. Eating vegetables instead of starchy carbs won't elevate your insulin levels. Almost every restaurant will happily accommodate this basic substitution any time, free of charge. All you have to do is ask.

2. Order an appetizer instead of eating from the basket of chips or bread.

Consider chips and bread to be nutritional land mines and avoid them at all costs. The solution: Eat something else. For instance, if you're ravenous when you sit down, right away order a side salad, an antipasto (it's the anti-pasta!), or a meat- or vegetable-only appetizer in order to avoid being tempted by the bottomless freebies. Also, choose salad over soup. Some soups are perfectly fine to eat, but for the most part, many have lots of hidden sugars and other foods that raise your insulin levels, shutting down your body's ability to burn fat.

3. Choose foods you eat with a fork, not with your fingers.

That means ordering beef, fish, or chicken that's served without buns or other types of bread. So sandwiches, wraps, and french fries are out, but steak is a great choice, as are fish and chicken when served without bread or breading. If you want a hamburger, simply discard the bun and eat it with a fork and knife. You might be accused of being a low-carb fanatic or even a sophisticate, but remember this: At any given time, you're either burning fat or storing fat. Your goal, of course, is to spend as much time in fat-burning mode as possible every day of your life. Leaving off the bread keeps your insulin and glycogen levels low, allowing you to do just that. Keep in mind that tortillas count as bread, too, so you'll want to avoid them even though we realize most people eat foods like burritos and enchiladas with a fork.

Frittata

Bacon

Sausage

Ham with melted cheese

Skirt steak

NexGen Muffins (page 96)

Halloumi Cheese (page 96)

Cream Cakes (page 97)

SNACKS

Cheese

Vegetables with ranch dressing

Nuts

Lunch meat

Pepperoni

Beef jerky

Boiled eggs

Pork rinds

Sugar-free Jell-O

Protein shakes

Leftovers from lunch and dinner

LUNCH AND DINNER

Steak Salad (page 98)

Taco Salad (page 100)

Tuna Salad (page 101)

Almond-Crusted Chicken (page 102)
  with Green Beans with Toasted Pine Nuts (page 103)

Chicken Curry (page 103)
  with Roasted Broccoli (page 104)

TNT TRANSFORMATION

"My back and shoulders widened, and my waist shrunk."

Name: **Jaimen Sanders**
Age: **19**
Height: **5 feet 8 inches**
Weight before: **243**
Weight after: **222**

JAIMEN SANDERS FIGURED HE HAD NOTHING TO LOSE by signing up for the TNT Diet study we were conducting at our University of Connecticut lab. But it turns out he was wrong: In just 12 weeks, Jaimen dropped 30 pounds of pure fat. And just as impressive, he added 9 pounds of new muscle at the same time.

"All my clothes suddenly started to fit better," says Jaimen, a student at UConn. "But the first change I noticed was having a lot more energy throughout the day. And I think both the diet and exercise allowed me to sleep less because I got better sleep at night." Interestingly, Jaimen found that sticking with the workout actually helped him stick to the diet. "The adrenaline rush and sensation of a completed workout kept me motivated. In fact, the exercise was probably the most fun part of the program besides the weekly weigh-ins."

All of which provides two lessons: First, that exercise can be just as important psychologically as it is physically. And second, that if you enjoy your workouts, you'll enjoy the results they help yield even more. After all, who wouldn't like weighing in, if, like Jaimen, you're losing 1 percent of your body fat a week? He also managed to drop his blood pressure from 150/95 to 128/86 and increased his HDL (good) cholesterol by 12 percent.

Because Jaimen had perhaps the best overall results we've ever witnessed on the TNT Diet (or any other plan, for that matter), we asked him the secrets of his success. Here they are:

- "Drink lots and lots of water. I always tried to have a glass before every meal."

- "Don't just rely on the scale to tell you how well you're doing. Pay more attention to how your body looks and feels, and how your clothes fit."

- "Don't quit after cheating. It'll happen once in a while, and that's okay; just hop right back on the plan. One of the best parts of the TNT Diet is that by not having sweets very often, they taste even better when you do have them. When I realized this, they became far less tempting on a daily basis."

Supplements That Work

While the TNT Diet is rich in vitamins, minerals, and antioxidants, no diet provides the optimal amount of all the nutrients you need. This is a not-so-well-known reality of human nutrition. For example, in one study, we analyzed the nutrient intake of people following either a low-carb or a low-fat diet. If a nutrient fell below 80 percent of the recommended dietary allowance (RDA), it was characterized as marginally deficient, whereas those less than 50 percent of the RDA were considered to be significantly deficient. The results:

	Low-Carb	Low-Fat
Marginally Deficient	Folate	Folate, calcium, magnesium, pantothenic acid
Significantly Deficient	Vitamin D, chromium	Zinc, vitamin D, vitamin E, chromium, molybdenum

These were just averages, of course. Nutrient intake can vary substantially from person to person depending on food preferences. A guy who eats several servings of vegetables a day will be far less likely to have a deficiency than one who doesn't down any.

That's why we believe that *everyone* should supplement their diet with a multivitamin, a recommendation that's endorsed by the American Medical Association. This ensures that all your nutritional bases are covered, which keeps you healthy and feeling energized.

Taking a daily multivitamin may even help prevent cancer. When researchers at the University of California starved human cells of vitamins and minerals, also called *micronutrients,* the resulting effect was DNA damage—a common culprit in deadly diseases like cancer. And even though most people's diets aren't dangerously deficient in vitamins and minerals, intakes are often inadequate. The result is that your body's stores of micronutrients are used for immediate needs instead of repairing damaged DNA, which would help preserve long-term health.

A once-daily multivitamin such as Centrum or Nature Made will help safeguard your DNA and shore up any nutritional holes in your diet. Just make sure to choose a men's formula that doesn't contain iron. Since you'll be eating lots of meat on the TNT Diet, you'll be downing all of this mineral that you need. Most products indicate if they're iron free on the front of the bottle, but your best strategy is to check the label to see if iron has been included.

The other supplement that we highly encourage you to take is fish oil. That's because fish oil is loaded with omega-3 fatty acids, healthy polyunsaturated fats that are essential for many biological functions. In dozens of studies, omega-3 fats have been shown to help prevent heart disease, as well as dozens of other afflictions.

A quick primer: There are several types of omega-3 fatty acids—the three main ones are eicosapentaenoic acid (EPA), docosahexaenoic acid (DHA), and alpha-linolenic acid (ALA). Don't worry about how to pronounce them; the acronyms are all you need to know.

EPA and DHA, the omega-3 fatty acids that are most easily used by your body, are found in significant amounts only in marine life, particularly cold-water fish (because they carry more fat for insulation). Of course, they're also found in the fish oil capsules that are created from these fish.

ALA, on the other hand, is obtained from plant-derived foods, such as flaxseed, canola oil, soybeans, pumpkin seeds, and walnuts. However, for ALA to provide health benefits, your liver must convert it into EPA and DHA. The estimated average efficiency of conversion is around 10 percent to 15 percent. That means for every gram of omega-3s you take in from fish sources, you need at least 6 grams from plant foods to glean an equivalent amount of EPA and DHA. The upshot: To provide your body with a healthy dose of omega-3 fats, you need to consume yours from either fish or fish oil. Trouble is, most Americans don't eat much fish, and even those who do would likely benefit from more. And that's where the capsules come in.

Thankfully, fish oil capsules appear to be every bit as effective as eating the fish itself. When researchers in Italy gave 2,800 heart attack survivors 1,000 milligrams of fish oil (composed almost entirely of EPA and DHA) a day, they found that the supplement reduced the risk of dying of heart disease by 30 percent and of sudden cardiac death by 45 percent, compared with those who didn't supplement their diets.

There's more:

- A British study found that when 70 depressed people consumed 1,000 milligrams of fish oil every day for 12 weeks, 69 percent of them experienced a 50 percent improvement in their symptoms. In addition, National Institutes of Health scientists determined that hostile, aggressive men have lower blood levels of DHA than their even-tempered counterparts, suggesting that increasing DHA may help with anger management issues.

- University of Pittsburgh researchers found that fish oil reduces chronic pain as well as ibuprofen and other nonsteroidal anti-inflammatory drugs (NSAIDs). When neck- and back-pain sufferers replaced their daily NSAID with 1,200 milligrams of fish oil for 10 weeks, 60 percent reported feeling better. In fact, 59 percent stopped taking their prescription NSAIDs altogether. Credit the twin powers of EPA and DHA, the essential fatty acids in fish oil that are converted to prostaglandins, compounds that fight inflammation.

- Other research shows that regular EPA and DHA consumption may lower the risk for colon cancer, stroke, asthma, arthritis, and dementia.

One warning: Not all fish oil provides the same amounts of EPA and DHA. Meaning, you'll find varying amounts of omega-3 fatty acids in 1,000 milligrams—a typical serving—of supplemental fish oil. The solution: Read the label. Aim for 1,000 milligrams to 2,000 milligrams a day of EPA and DHA combined (just add the amounts together), whether that means one capsule or three. You can take more, but unless your doctor advises it because of a medical condition, cap your intake at 3,000 milligrams a day. Because fish oil acts as a blood thinner, some experts believe that taking it in high amounts—more than 3,000 milligrams of EPA and DHA per day—could result in excessive bleeding if you're in a serious accident. (It's not a major concern; just consider it our obligatory disclaimer.)

Our favorite brand: Nordic Naturals Ultra Omega, which is available at www.nordicnaturals.com. One serving (two capsules) of these odorless, nearly tasteless gel capsules provides 650 milligrams EPA and 450 milligrams DHA—for a total of 1,100 milligrams of healthy omega-3 fatty acids.

CHAPTER 6

THE RELOADING TIME ZONE

When you think of the Reloading Time Zone, just imagine your muscles literally filling up with nutrients. You'll not only be able to feel your muscles become tighter and fuller, you'll probably notice the changes in the mirror. Why? Because you'll be replenishing your glycogen stores by eating a hefty dose of carbohydrates. At the same time, this influx of carbs will raise your insulin levels, which drives even more nutrients—such as the high-quality protein that you eat—to your muscles. The result is a dramatic surge in muscle growth. And even better, all of this occurs without causing your body to store fat. The reason: Whenever you enter the Reloading Time Zone, your glycogen levels will be low, due to the time you've spent in the Fat-Burning Time Zone. This prepares your body to embrace high-carb foods, without the negative consequences that occur when your glycogen tank is overflowing.

You'll probably notice that many of the Reloading Time Zone foods are similar to those in the Fat-Burning Time Zone. For instance, meat, cheese, and eggs are all excellent sources of muscle-building protein, which makes them ideal for both Time Zones. However, since there's no need to watch your carb intake in the Reloading Time Zone, the approved list of high-quality protein sources expands to include yogurt, kefir, and milk. The same goes for produce: In addition to the options you have in the Fat-Burning Zone, you can now eat as much fruit as you want and add starchy vegetables such as potatoes, carrots, and corn to your meals.

The main change between the Fat-Burning Time Zone and the Reloading Time Zone is that you'll now emphasize healthy, high-carbohydrate foods, such as grains and beans, and de-emphasize foods that are high in fat. But again, the key is to keep the diet simple. And you can do just that by following the nutrition tactics below.

THE NUTRITION TACTICS

1. Eat any combination of the Reloading Time Zone foods—along with the approved condiments and beverages—until you feel satisfied, but not stuffed. Again, don't overthink this; just eat. By following the general guidelines that we've laid out here, you'll automatically avoid junk food, the universal downfall of all diets.

2. Try to eat high-quality protein at every meal and every 3 hours, if possible. The goal is to provide your muscles with a steady supply of amino acids, in order to ensure that they have the nutrients they need to grow. Think of it as if you were constructing a new house: If you don't have all of the necessary building materials on hand, even the best builder can't make progress.

3. Consume carbohydrates at each meal. This shouldn't be too hard, since it's in line with the way most people are accustomed to eating. The idea is to boost your insulin levels at every meal, in order to drive nutrients to your muscles. So during the Reloading Time Zone, besides vegetables, you can enjoy pasta, sandwiches, cereal, and pancakes, as well as snacks such as fruit, popcorn, and pretzels.

4. Go easy on extra fats. The reason is simple: You can only eat so many calories in a day without gaining fat. And since you'll be increasing your intake of carbs, that doesn't leave a lot of room for additional calories from sources such as nuts, seeds, and butter. This doesn't mean you should eliminate fat altogether, only that your intake should be incidental. So limit your diet to the fat that's naturally found in meat or cheese, or the kind needed to cook with, like olive oil.

5. Avoid added sugar and refined grains. Primarily, this means foods that are made with sugar—regular soda, cake, cookies—or with flour that isn't 100 percent whole wheat, like white bread and white pasta. Technically, these carbohydrates are allowed in the Reloading Time Zone, when the purpose is to raise insulin levels. However, we highly encourage you to eat *quality* sources of carbohydrates. That is, carb-rich foods that are also packed with nutrients, such as 100 percent whole grain products and high-fiber beans. These are what we call nutrient-dense carbohydrates.

THE RELOADING TIME ZONE FOODS

HIGH-QUALITY PROTEIN	FRUITS AND VEGETABLES*		NUTRIENT-DENSE CARBOHYDRATES
Beef	Asparagus	Apples	Beans
Cheese	Broccoli	Bananas	Bread
Eggs and egg whites	Carrots	Berries	Cereal
Fish	Corn	Grapes	Flour
Kefir	Onions	Melon	Oats
Milk	Peppers	Oranges	Pasta
Pork	Potatoes	Peaches	Quinoa
Poultry	Spinach	Pears	Rice
Yogurt	Tomatoes	Pineapple	Tortillas

*These are just a few common examples of fruits and vegetables; just about any type of produce imaginable is acceptable.

HIGH-QUALITY PROTEIN

This category is the same as in the Fat-Burning Time Zone, but with three additions: milk, yogurt, and kefir. Also, you may now choose any type of cheese, including cottage cheese and ricotta. For the best results, follow these guidelines:

• Choose lean cuts of beef, such as 90 to 95 percent lean ground beef. While cooking, feel free to substitute egg whites for whole eggs. Remember, this isn't to suggest that fat is bad, only that when you're eating lots of carbohydrates in the Reloading Time Zone, you should limit your fat intake—and this is a simple way to do it.

• When you have a choice, opt for the fat-free or 2% versions of cheese, milk, yogurt, and kefir. This is just the opposite of the Fat-Burning Time Zone, when full-fat products are the default. However, don't feel like you need to buy, for example, full-fat Cheddar cheese for the Fat-Burning Time Zone, and reduced-fat Cheddar for the Reloading Time Zone. That will likely result in not only a higher grocery bill but also waste, since the duration of the Reloading Time Zone is short. In that case, go ahead and have the full-fat version. But go reduced-fat when it makes sense—like when you buy individual containers of yogurt.

What Is Kefir?

Similar to yogurt, this fermented dairy beverage is made by culturing fresh milk with kefir grains.

Why it's healthy: Because kefir contains gut-friendly bacteria, it's been shown to lower cholesterol, improve lactose digestion, and enhance the immune system. In addition, University of Washington scientists recently demonstrated that kefir is more effective at helping people control hunger than fruit juice.

Where to find it: Look for kefir in the health food section of your local super-market, or in the dairy aisle of health food stores, such as Whole Foods.

• Although the flavored versions of milk, yogurt, and kefir are all accept-able—such as chocolate milk or fruit-on-the-bottom yogurt—they often contain high amounts of added sugars. Case in point: A cup of Colombo blueberry yogurt packs 36 grams of sugar, only about half of which is found naturally in the yogurt and fruit. The rest comes in the form of "added" sugar—or what we prefer to call "unnecessary." Does this mean you can't have chocolate milk or fruit-on-the-bottom yogurt? Not at all. We're just advising you that these aren't the very *healthiest* options. In terms of body composition, though, they won't affect your results at all. And in fact, you'll find that chocolate milk and kefir are excellent choices in the Muscle-Building Time Zone, if you're following the Protein + Carbohydrates recommendations for TNT Plan B, D, or E.

FRUITS AND VEGETABLES

For the Reloading Time Zone, we can't think of a fruit or vegetable that you shouldn't eat. We've provided a short list below, but in general, eat as much produce as you desire—even if it's not on the list.

A few additional details:

• Choose from fresh, frozen, and canned products that contain no added sugars. Just check the ingredient list: The only item listed should be the fruit or vegetable itself.

• Add fruit and vegetable juices to your drink list. In addition to the TNT-approved beverages in Chapter 8, you can also have juice in the Reloading Time Zone. Choose only products that are 100 percent fruit or vegetable juice, though. Again, the only ingredients listed should be the juice from the fruits or vegetables themselves.

THE RELOADING TIME ZONE-APPROVED VEGETABLES

Alfalfa sprouts	Cauliflower	Mushrooms	Spaghetti squash
Artichokes	Celery	Okra	Spinach
Arugula	Corn	Onions	Summer squash
Asparagus	Cucumber	Peppers (any color)	Sweet potatoes
Bean sprouts	Eggplant	Potatoes	Tomatoes
Bok choy	Endive	Radishes	Turnips
Broccoli	Green beans	Sauerkraut	Watercress
Brussels sprouts	Kale	Scallions	Zucchini
Carrots	Lettuce (any type)	Snow peas	

• Easy does it on the dried fruit. Sure, it's a great Reloading Time Zone snack: Per ½ cup, dried fruit packs substantially more disease-fighting antioxidants than its fresh counterpart. That's because it's been dehydrated—which sucks out the water, but not the nutrients. This makes each piece smaller, giving you more total pieces than in a comparable serving

THE RELOADING TIME ZONE-APPROVED FRUITS

Apples	Cranberries	Peaches
Apricots	Grapefruit	Pears
Bananas	Grapes	Pineapple
Blackberries	Honeydew melon	Plums
Blueberries	Kiwifruit	Raspberries
Boysenberries	Mangoes	Strawberries
Cantaloupe	Nectarines	Tangerines
Cherries	Oranges	Watermelon

of fresh fruit. But dried fruit also packs significantly more calories and is far sweeter. (It tastes more like candy than fruit.) All of which makes it an easy snack to overindulge on. Your rule of thumb: If you choose to eat dried fruit, limit yourself to one to two handfuls a day, just to be safe.

NUTRIENT-DENSE CARBOHYDRATES

Here's the reality: In the Reloading Time Zone, it really doesn't matter what type of carbohydrates you eat. At least not in terms of how much fat you lose or how much muscle you build. That's because, eventually, carbohydrates in the form of sugar and starch are all broken down into sugar in your digestive tract. (See "Carbohydrates . . . Explained" on page 64.) So to some extent, your body doesn't know the difference between the carbohydrates in a slice of whole grain bread and those found in a piece of angel food cake. Both will fill your glycogen tank equally well and raise your insulin levels, which is what you want to do to create a surge of muscle growth.

However, we're concerned with more than just body composition. To achieve the maximum benefit for your health, we advise that you limit your consumption of added sugars—those that aren't found naturally in a food—because they have no other nutritional value. Likewise, the same can be said for foods that are high in starch but low in fiber and other nutrients—such as refined grains as opposed to whole grains.

Our philosophy is that choosing "whole foods" is the best approach because they usually come with a healthy dose of vitamins, minerals, antioxidants, and other natural anti-inflammatories. These nutrients can help ward off disease, give you more energy to train, and ensure that you have less downtime due to illness. Think of a high-performance racing car: It can run on basic 87-octane fuel, but you'll get more horsepower from the engine if you feed it cleaner 93-octane fuel. The same can be said for your body and the food you eat. When you consume carbohydrates from added sugars and refined grains that have little nutritional value—other than simply providing carbohydrates—you're essentially putting cheap gas in your high-performance body.

For that reason, we focus on "nutrient-dense" carbohydrates. These are carbohydrates derived from sources that are closest to the way they're found in nature—for example, you should always choose bread made with 100 percent whole wheat flour instead of white flour, which has been highly processed and stripped of valuable nutrients.

Now does that mean you can't enjoy a piece of cake or a bag of gummy bears in the Reloading Time Zone? No, it just means those aren't the optimal choices for your health. The truth is, the Reloading Time Zone is the best time for you to "cheat" on the diet (see "The TNT Guide to Cheating" below). But because we have to live with ourselves, we're going to tell you how to make the healthiest food choices; the rest is up to you.

HOW TO MAKE THE BEST CARB CHOICES

1. Choose 100 percent whole grain bread, pasta, and rice. This includes bread products, such as bagels, tortillas, and English muffins. Don't be fooled by products—often breakfast cereals—that just state, "Made with whole grains." This claim simply means that at least 51 percent of the flour it's made with is from a whole grain source. But the rest of the flour can come from refined grains—and likely does. If it's really "100 percent whole grain," it usually says so on the package. Check the ingredient list: Any flour that doesn't start with the word "whole" isn't. And it's either whole grain rice or it isn't. Also, ingredients are listed in descending order of the amount used.

The TNT Guide to Cheating

Full disclosure: Because the objective of the Reloading Time Zone is to replenish glycogen and raise insulin levels, it's the absolute best time for you to indulge your cravings for junk foods such as candy, chips, regular soda, and even take-out pizza. Again, we don't recommend these foods for your health, or for optimal results. But we do realize that most people won't follow the guidelines of this diet—or any other diet—100 percent of the time. So by limiting all intake of these foods to the Reloading Time Zone—when your glycogen levels are low—you'll be able to eat them without significantly sabotaging your progress. This strategy also ensures that you're eating healthy foods *most* of the time.

All of this is provided, of course, that you don't overdo it. After all, junk foods are high in calories and taste good, which means they're easy to overeat. Down too much of them, and you'll fill your glycogen tank, priming your body to store fat. Sure, you could overeat whole grains, beans, fruits, and vegetables, too, but it's not likely—especially in the duration of the Reloading Time Zone. So as a general guideline, limit junk foods to one meal during the Reloading Time Zone. For instance, that might mean a take-out pizza night for one guy, and "lunch" at an ice cream shop for another.

2. Opt for products that have the fewest ingredients. As a general guideline, this is one of the best ways to choose foods. Think about it: A vegetable or a piece of fruit has only one ingredient—why shouldn't you strive for the rest of your carbohydrates to meet that criteria?

Carbohydrates . . . Explained

Throughout this book, you've read a lot about carbohydrates. But you might still be wondering: What exactly are they? The simple answer is sugar, starch, and fiber. Which, of course, leads to three more questions:

What's sugar? The most basic types of sugar are: glucose, which is the form of sugar your body uses for energy; fructose, which is found naturally in fruit and honey; and galactose, which combines with glucose to form lactose, the sugar that gives milk its sweetness. However, when most people talk about sugar, they're typically referring to sucrose, or table sugar. Table sugar is composed of nearly equal parts of two simple sugars, glucose and fructose. Since glucose circulates in your bloodstream, it's already in the form your body needs. So it's easily digested and quickly raises blood sugar and insulin. Fructose, however, has to be processed in your liver, where it's either converted to fat or to glucose. This slows down the rate that it's digested, and reduces its impact on your blood sugar.

What's starch? Remember how glycogen is your body's stored glucose? Well, starch is a plant's stored glucose. In fact, think of starch—the primary carbohydrate in bread, rice, pasta, and other flour-based foods—as a bundle of glucose molecules, held together by weak chemical bonds. These bonds start to dissolve the moment they make contact with saliva, immediately freeing the glucose to be absorbed into your bloodstream. So to your body, starch is simply a hefty dose of sugar in the form of glucose. As a result, starch has an even greater impact on blood sugar than sucrose.

What's fiber? Fiber is the structural material of plants, which is found in their stems, leaves, roots, and skins. It's known as a "nonavailable" carbohydrate because humans can't break it down for energy. So in a sense, it fills your belly without providing calories. (Fiber does contain calories, but your body can't access them.) Our inability to digest fiber is why people often talk about "net" carbs: It refers to the total amount of carbohydrates in a food, minus the fiber, since, practically speaking, it doesn't count. The satiety fiber gives is one reason why whole grain bread is better than white bread, which has been stripped of its fiber and other nutrients through processing. (See "From the Field to Flour" on page 66.)

3. If it has added sugars, skip it. How can you tell? Read the Nutrition Facts label and look under "carbohydrates" for "sugars." If the food doesn't contain any fruit or milk (which contain natural sugars) but has sugar, then they've added it to sweeten the product. Again, check the ingredient list: Does it list sugar of any kind? (See "Sugar by Any Other Name . . ." on page 39 for a complete list of sugars.) Mostly, though, by avoiding the foods that you know you shouldn't be eating in the first place—regular soda, candy, baked goods, ice cream—you'll cut out most of the added sugar in your diet.

GRAINS

For the most part, this food group includes any grain or product made from grains, including bread, pasta, rice, and flour. (Include quinoa in this category, too; you'll find a complete user's guide on page 72.) To make it easier for you to navigate the grocery store aisles, we've selected our favorite products in several categories.

The Best Breads

Food for Life Ezekiel 4:9 Sprouted Whole Grain Products

Bread

Hamburger buns

What's Sprouted Grain Bread?

Sprouted grain bread is made when fresh grains and legumes such as wheat, barley, beans, oats, spelt, and millet are allowed to sprout, instead of being ground into flour. Then the sprouts are formed into batches of dough and slowly baked. Products created from sprouted grains have more essential protein, fiber, and B vitamins than those made with refined flour, according to research conducted in India.

Where to find it: Because it has no preservatives, this bread must be kept frozen. Look for the most widely available brand—Food for Life Ezekiel 4:9—in the freezer aisle of your grocery store's health food section.

English muffins

Pocket breads

Tortillas

Why we chose them: These products have no preservatives and are made with 100 percent whole grains. Although they're harder to find than many other commercial brands, they're the healthiest breads we've found. Go to www.foodforlife.com to locate a store near you. Also, as a close runner-up, we highly recommend the products from Alvarado Street Bakery, which are available in many health food stores and online (www.alvaradostreetbakery.com).

From the Field to Flour

Did you ever wonder how far removed a piece of bread is from a kernel of wheat? Here's an insider's look, courtesy of Kendall McFall, a flour-milling instructor at Kansas State University.

1. A combine harvests wheat from the fields and removes the whole grain kernels from the stalks. The kernels are then transported to the mill.

2. At the mill, corrugated rollers break open the kernel and scrape the carb-loaded endosperm away from the bran—the high-fiber outer husk—and the vitamin-rich germ, which is the embryo of the kernel.

3. After the rollers pulverize all parts of the grain kernel, they're fed through sifters, which separate the larger bran and germ particles from the endosperm.

4. The bran and germ are routed into different machines for further processing while heavy rollers smooth the remaining endosperm fragments into a fine powder, or flour.

5A. For refined flour: The grain kernel flour is enriched—as mandated by federal law—with thiamine, niacin, riboflavin, folic acid, and iron. The flour may also be bleached at this point, before being packaged.

5B. For whole wheat flour: The powdered endosperm, bran, and germ particles are recombined in the same proportion as were present in the whole kernel. This flour is not enriched.

6. The flour is packaged and ready to be made into bread.

—Reporting by Heather Loeb

The Best Pasta
Barilla Plus

Why we chose it: It's made with high-fiber flax flour, which contains heart-healthy omega-3 fatty acids. Make sure that "Plus" is included in the product name, as regular Barilla pasta is made from refined flour. Also, 100 percent whole wheat couscous—which is actually the grain from which pasta flour is made—is a great alternative.

The Best Rice
Uncle Ben's Fast & Natural Whole Grain Instant Brown Rice

Why we chose it: Besides being quick and easy to prepare, it has one ingredient—whole grain rice. Any 100 percent whole grain rice product is acceptable, though, including basmati.

The Best Tortillas
MexAmerica Whole Wheat Flour Tortillas

Why we chose them: One of the few tortilla brands made with whole wheat flour that can also be found in most grocery stores. Food for Life Ezekiel 4:9 sprouted grain tortillas are a good choice, too, but are less flexible—which makes them good for quesadillas, but not so good for wraps.

The Best Bagels
Thomas' Hearty Grains 100% Whole Wheat Bagel

Why we chose them: They taste good, and they meet the 100 percent whole wheat standard. Look for them in your grocery store's bakery section, not the freezer.

The Best Slow-Cook Oatmeal
Bob's Red Mill Steel-Cut Oats

Why we chose them: Steel-cut oats are not as processed as the more common rolled oats. They also have a nuttier, chewier taste. Plus, this brand contains no added sugar. They're simply the inside of the oat kernel, cut into two or three coarse pieces. For comparison, the more popular rolled oats are pieces of the inner oat kernel that have been steamed, rolled, and then steamed again, in order to create a thin oat "flake."

The Best Instant Oatmeal
Nature's Path Organic Instant Hot Oatmeal (Original)

Why we chose it: The ingredient list, which reads: "Organic rolled oats, sea salt." Note that the flavored varieties in the Nature's Path line all contain at least one other ingredient—"organic evaporated cane juice." In other words, added sugar, which is the norm for any brand of flavored oatmeal.

The Best Crackers
Triscuit Original Wheat Crackers

Why we chose them: All things considered, it's not a bad product. It's made with 100 percent whole wheat, oil, and salt.

Beans
This category is simple: We recommend all types of beans with one caveat—the baked variety. That's because baked beans are typically covered in a sauce made with brown and white sugars. Consider that 1 cup of canned baked beans contains 24 grams of sugar—about the same amount in 8 ounces of regular soda. So they're not the best choice. Keep in mind that besides black beans, kidney beans, navy beans, white beans, and lima beans—among others—this food group also includes hummus.

Cereal
Our criteria for choosing cereals is easy: Look for products that are made with 100 percent whole grains and don't contain any added sugar. Sugar from fruit is acceptable, but if it's simply being used as a sweetener, skip it. Since

these stipulations disqualify 95 percent of the cereals in your supermarket, we sifted through the aisles for you to find the very best choices.

Food for Life Ezekiel 4:9 Sprouted Grain Cereal

Where to find: The health food section of your grocery store

Flavors: Original; Golden Flax; Almond; Cinnamon Raisin

Bear Naked All Natural Low Sugar Cereal

Where to find: The health food section of your grocery store. For more information, go to www.bearnakedgranola.com/cereal.htm

Flavors: Triple Berry Crunch; Vanilla Almond Crunch

General Mills Fiber One Bran Cereal

Where to find: The main cereal aisle of your grocery store

Flavor: Original

Post Shredded Wheat Cereal

Where to find: The main cereal aisle of your grocery store

Flavor: Original

RELOADING TIME ZONE-APPROVED CONDIMENTS, SPICES, AND HERBS

Just about every condiment, spice, or herb you could want is acceptable in the Reloading Time Zone, including ketchup and barbecue sauce. We do recommend that you avoid mayonnaise, aioli, and creamy salad dressings (blue cheese, ranch, Thousand Island) when possible, though, since they fall under the category of "added fats."

THE RELOADING TIME ZONE MENU

Here are some examples of the foods you can have for breakfast, lunch, dinner, and snacks. Just like in the Fat-Burning Zone, this is just a sampling of the meals you might eat at certain times of the day. The only true guidelines are the Reloading Time Zone Nutrition Tactics that were presented at the beginning of this chapter. Remember, the idea is that you focus on the foods themselves, not the quantity.

BREAKFAST

Cereal with milk and fruit

Whole wheat toast

Oatmeal with fruit

Quinoa (page 72)

Pancakes

Waffles

Yogurt and fruit

Turkey sausage

Scrambled eggs or egg whites

Omelet or egg-white omelet

- Denver
- Greek
- Ham and cheese
- Western
- Any other combination of meats, vegetables, and cheeses

SNACKS

Vegetables

Fruit

Popcorn

Pretzels

Milk

100 percent fruit juice

Yogurt

Protein shake

Leftovers from lunch and dinner

LUNCH AND DINNER

Sausage and Red Pepper Pizza (page 116)

Tuna Salad Sandwich (page 101)

Deli sandwich

Hamburger

Grilled chicken sandwich

Peppers with Quinoa Stuffing (page 74)

Pasta

- Penne Puttanesca with Chicken (page 110)
- Meatballs (page 123) with spaghetti
- Sausage with Feta and Spinach (page 114) with pasta
- Just about any type of pasta that you like

Kielbasa and Lentil Soup (page 115)

Burritos (page 128)

Chicken Stir-Fry (page 105) over brown rice

Breaded Chicken (page 102)

Beef Kebabs (page 118)
  with Quinoa Salad (page 73)

Rosemary Pork Tenderloin (page 113)
  with Quinoa Risotto (page 75)

Taco Salad (page 100)

Roasted Chicken (page 108)

Cilantro Flank Steak (page 119)
  with sweet potato

Steak Salad (page 98)

The User's Guide to Quinoa

If you're like most guys, you've never even heard of quinoa (pronounced "keen-wah"). That's a shame because it's one of the healthiest grains you can eat. Check that: Quinoa is technically classified as a seed, but its nutrient profile is so similar to that of a grain that it's often confused for one. Regardless, it provides something that's rare among plant foods: Like meat, eggs, and dairy, quinoa packs all nine of the essential amino acids that your body needs to build muscle. That makes it a high-quality protein. And because it's also packed with carbohydrates, it may be the ideal Reloading Time Zone food.

Quinoa has an addictive nutty flavor, cooks up quicker than brown rice, and can be used to make stuffings, risottos, and salads. The downside: Few guys know where to find it, let alone how to prepare it. But typically, you can locate quinoa in the rice aisle, or the health food section of your grocery store. You can also stock up on it at www.edenfoods.com.

Before cooking, place the quinoa in a strainer and rinse thoroughly. This will remove any residue of saponin, a bitter substance that covers the outside of the seed and that turns soapy in water. (Typically, prepackaged quinoa has already been rinsed, but it's best to give it a quick wash anyway.)

As for preparation, the simplest way is to cook quinoa like pasta: Fill a large pot or saucepan with water and bring to a boil. Add just about any amount of quinoa, turn the heat to low, and cook until tender, about 20 minutes. Drain and allow the quinoa to cool. Cook up a big batch, store it in an airtight container in your refrigerator (you can keep it for up to a week), and you'll have a ready-to-eat side dish that goes with just about any meal. (Just microwave for 1 to 2 minutes to warm.)

Even better, we asked our good friend and *Men's Health* resident chef Matt Goulding to provide the recipes and tweaks that follow so that you can turn this simple grain into more than a dozen dishes.

Quinoa Breakfast

Combine 1 cup cooked quinoa with ½ cup milk and ½ cup frozen blueberries and microwave for 60 seconds. This makes a great alternative to oatmeal.

Quinoa Salad

8   spears asparagus

1½   teaspoons olive oil plus a drizzle for the asparagus
     Salt

1   cup quinoa, cooked as directed on page 72

¼   cup olives, pitted and coarsely chopped

¼   cup chopped sundried tomatoes

2   ounces crumbled goat cheese or feta cheese

1   tablespoon balsamic or red wine vinegar
     Pepper

1. Preheat the oven to 400°F. Remove the woody ends from the asparagus by gently bending each spear until it breaks—it will naturally snap off at the right place. Lay on a cookie sheet or baking pan, drizzle with olive oil, sprinkle with a pinch of salt, and toss. Roast for 10 minutes.

2. Chop the asparagus into bite-size pieces. In a bowl, combine the asparagus, quinoa, olives, sundried tomatoes, cheese, vinegar, and 1½ teaspoons olive oil. Season with salt and pepper to taste.

Change It Up

For other great salads, try mixing cooked quinoa with any of the following combinations:

- A sliced avocado, the segments of 1 grapefruit, a handful of chopped green onions, and the juice of half a lime. Great with grilled fish.

- ½ cup dried cranberries, ¼ cup chopped walnuts, a handful of crumbled blue cheese, and 1 tablespoon each balsamic vinegar and olive oil.

- 2 cups baby spinach or arugula, 8 ounces grilled chicken, and ¼ cup roasted red peppers.

Peppers with Quinoa Stuffing

- 1 teaspoon olive oil
- ½ yellow onion, chopped
- 2 Roma tomatoes, seeded and chopped
- 2 cloves garlic, minced
- 6 ounces shrimp, peeled and deveined
- ½ cup canned black beans, drained and rinsed
- ½ teaspoon cumin
- ½ cup quinoa, cooked as directed on page 72
-    Handful chopped fresh cilantro
-    Salt and pepper to taste
- 2 red bell peppers

1. Preheat the oven to 400°F. Heat the olive oil in a sauté pan over medium heat. Add the onion, tomatoes, and garlic and cook until the tomato is soft and the onion is translucent, about 3 minutes. Add the shrimp, beans, and cumin and cook for another 3 minutes, until the shrimp is just pink and firm. Add the cooked quinoa and cilantro, stir to blend, and remove from heat. Season with salt and pepper.

2. Cut the tops off the peppers and remove the ribs and seeds. Stuff each with half of the mixture. Place in a baking pan and bake 15 minutes.

Change It Up

- Replace the shrimp, cumin, and cilantro with 2 links chicken sausage and a 6-ounce jar of marinated artichoke hearts.

- Replace the shrimp with 8 ounces lean ground beef or ground turkey.

- Go Greek: Trade the shrimp, cilantro, cumin, and black beans for lean ground beef, 1 cup frozen spinach, and ½ cup crumbled feta cheese.

Quinoa Risotto

1 teaspoon olive oil

1 medium yellow onion, diced

2 cloves garlic, minced

1 cup uncooked quinoa

3 cups low-sodium chicken stock

¼ cup fresh or frozen peas

2 ounces prosciutto, cut into thin strips

Salt and pepper to taste

Parmesan cheese for grating

1. Heat the olive oil in a medium sauté or saucepan over medium heat and add the onion and garlic. Cook until the onion is translucent, about 3 minutes.

2. Add the quinoa and cook for another 3 minutes. Add 1 cup of the chicken stock, using a wooden spoon to occasionally stir the grains. When the liquid has mostly evaporated (about 10 minutes), add the remaining stock. Continue cooking and stirring until the quinoa is tender (but not mushy) and most of the liquid has evaporated; the risotto should be moist, but not soupy. At the last minute, add the peas and prosciutto and stir to warm through.

3. Remove from heat; season with salt and pepper. Before serving, grate a bit of Parmesan over each portion.

Change It Up

- Replace the peas and prosciutto with 1 cup shredded rotisserie chicken (or leftover grilled chicken), 1 cup cherry tomatoes, and a handful of chopped fresh basil.

- Add ½ pound sliced mushrooms to the pan with the onion and garlic. Before adding the stock, add ½ cup red wine. Peas and prosciutto are optional.

- Replace the peas and prosciutto with ½ cup canned pumpkin puree. Stir in a handful of chopped fresh sage a few seconds before you remove from the heat. Great with pork tenderloin.

"I cut my body-fat percentage in half."

Name: **Jean-Paul (J.P.) Francoeur**
Age: **38**
Height: **5 feet 8 inches**
Weight before: **202**
Weight after: **175**

J.P. FRANCOEUR HAD FINALLY HAD ENOUGH: His body-fat percentage had just hit 22 percent, a measure that classified him as overweight. And although that's far from unusual these days, it made him dread going to work.

Why? Because J.P. is a personal trainer—has been for 17 years—and the owner of one of the top health clubs in Little Rock, Arkansas. "One of the most important things a trainer can do is look the part," says J.P. "I didn't."

And at the time, he was also the chairman of the Arkansas Governor's Council on Fitness. In fact, he even had a hand in Governor Mike Huckabee's widely publicized 100-pound weight loss.

So how come he couldn't help himself? His story may sound familiar: Over the previous couple of years, a hectic lifestyle had led to poor eating habits and skipped workouts. "I'm on the go 12 hours a day trying to run the business, then I have 3 hours of mayhem at home trying to keep up with three kids," says J.P. "Who has time to count calories and fill out food journals?"

That's when he decided to try the TNT Diet which provided the no-hassle program he needed. "In the first 8 weeks, I lost 20 pounds, and my performance in the gym not only didn't suffer as it does on most diets, it improved." Even better, J.P.'s body-fat percentage dropped from 22 percent to 14 percent, and then down to 11 percent a few weeks later. "The best part is that I never felt hungry, and I was eating more healthy vegetables than ever before," explains J.P. "The downside? I had to go out and buy all new clothes."

CHAPTER 7

THE MUSCLE-BUILDING TIME ZONE

I f you want to get the most from your workout—and who doesn't?—you should never again think of diet and exercise separately. Instead, you should adopt the mindset that they actually *depend* on each other. After all, lifting weights signals your body to build muscle, but you still need to eat the right nutrients—the Muscle-Building Time Zone foods—to provide your muscles with the raw materials for growth. And likewise, simply eating the Muscle-Building Time Zone foods won't add inches to your chest, arms, and shoulders, if you aren't regularly pumping iron.

But there's one more key factor involved, besides just eating the right foods and doing the right kind of exercise: timing. With the exception of bodybuilders, few people ever think about what they eat in the time before or after their workout. That's unfortunate because it's the period when nutrition strategies can have the most dramatic effect on muscle growth. To fully understand why workout nutrition has such a huge impact, you'll need the accompanying quick lesson in "The Science of Muscle Growth" (page 79). Once you grasp the basics of building muscle, you have the power to accelerate muscle growth with food. How? Two ways:

1. Eat protein. This boosts the level of amino acids in your blood. These amino acids—which are the building blocks of protein—travel through your body to wherever they're needed. Once they arrive at, say, your muscles, individual amino acids group together, or *synthesize,* to form the new proteins needed to build muscle. Research shows that as blood levels of amino acids rise, so does your rate of protein synthesis. The best part: This has no effect on your body's ability to use fat for energy. Protein in your diet—consumed in coordination with your workout—can give you high-powered muscle growth while your body continues to burn blubber.

2. Eat carbohydrates. This increases your insulin levels, which signals your body to stop using stored protein for energy. The upshot:

It decreases protein breakdown. Of course, if your glycogen levels are full, the insulin surge will signal your body to stop burning—and start storing—fat. But if your glycogen levels aren't full? You'll still be burning fat, although it won't be at the same maximal rate that occurs when you eat protein only.

Now, if it isn't obvious, the best way to stimulate maximum muscle growth is to consume both protein and carbohydrates during the period immediately before or after your workout. However, if you're more concerned with maximum fat loss, then just eating protein is the best approach. We've provided strategies for each.

The Muscle-Building Time Zone starts 1 hour before your workout and lasts until 30 minutes after your training session. Your primary task during this time is to consume the vital amount of nutrients needed to take full advantage of this muscle-building window of opportunity. We'll show you how, but first note that there are two different categories of foods in the Muscle-Building Time Zone that you can select from: One that provides only high-quality protein (Protein Only) and one that supplies both protein and carbohydrates (Protein + Carbohydrates). Simply opt for the category that matches the TNT Plan that you've chosen to follow. A reminder:

- TNT Plan A: Protein Only
- TNT Plan B: Protein + Carbohydrates
- TNT Plan C: Protein Only
- TNT Plan D: Protein + Carbohydrates
- TNT Plan E: Protein + Carbohydrates

(If you haven't yet determined which plan is right for you, flip back to page 25 and do so now.)

THE NUTRITION TACTICS

Follow the guidelines for the specific Muscle-Building Time Zone category—Protein Only or Protein + Carbohydrates—that corresponds to your TNT Plan. In either category, do your best to adhere to the "ideal" protocol when possible. This strategy is the optimal nutrition tactic to employ in the Muscle-Building Time Zone. Of course, depending on when you work out, your schedule, and your budget, you may find this isn't always practical. So your primary objective is to, at the very least, abide by the "practical alternatives" guidelines. Don't worry; this alternative provides you with most of the benefits that accompany smart workout nutrition.

THE MUSCLE-BUILDING TIME ZONE: PROTEIN ONLY (PLANS A AND C)

THE IDEAL

● Prepare a protein shake (made with water) that provides at least 40 grams of whey and/or casein protein. When choosing a product, look for one that contains only small amounts of carbs and fat. Here are three products we like, but comparable protein powders work as well. Keep in mind that if the product provides, say, 24 grams of protein per serving, you'll want to have two servings. Of course, that'll result in 48 grams of protein, which is absolutely fine. Remember, your charge is to consume a *minimum* of 40 grams.

The Science of Muscle Growth

The more protein your body stores—through protein synthesis—the larger your muscles grow. In fact, just as glycogen is stored carbohydrate, and belly fat is, well, stored fat, muscle is actually stored protein. (Protein is stored other places as well, like joints and ligaments.)

However, your body is constantly draining your protein reserves for other uses, such as energy, or to make hormones. This is known as protein breakdown, and it's happening all throughout the day. So to build muscle, you need to store new proteins faster than your body breaks down old proteins. You can do this by either increasing protein synthesis or decreasing protein breakdown, or, of course, by doing both.

Interestingly, research shows that, in guys who lift weights after an overnight fast, resistance training increases protein breakdown (bad) even more than it boosts protein synthesis (good). That means lifting weights doesn't result in more muscle if you don't eat. And though most of us don't skip meals for 10 to 12 hours before and after exercise, it's important to understand that protein breakdown is elevated for up to 48 hours after a hard workout. This is where the Muscle-Building Time Zone comes in.

- ProSource NytroWhey Extreme (2 servings)—this is the same protein powder used in our most recent study

   Available at: www.prosource.net

   Per serving: 22 grams protein, 1 gram carbohydrate, zero gram fat

- Biotest Metabolic Drive Super Protein Shake (2 servings)

   Available at: www.t-nation.com

   Per serving: 20 grams protein, 4 grams carbohydrate, 1½ grams fat

- At Large Nutrition Nitrean (2 servings)

   Available at: www.atlargenutrition.com

   Per serving: 24 grams protein, 2 grams carbohydrate, 1 gram fat

- Drink half of the beverage 30 to 45 minutes before your workout; drink the other half immediately after your workout.

- Eat a Fat-Burning Time Zone meal or snack that contains high-quality protein within 30 minutes to 1 hour after your training session. (Your snack could be another 20- to 40-gram protein shake.)

PRACTICAL ALTERNATIVES

Good: Consume at least 20 grams of high-quality protein, in the form of solid food, 45 to 60 minutes before your workout. Then eat a regular meal (Fat-Burning Time Zone) within 1 hour after your training session. The best choices for pre-workout protein:

- 1 small can (3½ ounces) tuna

- 3 to 4 ounces (3 to 4 slices) lean deli meat, such as turkey or chicken

- 1 serving of any kind of lean meat that's about the size (length, width, and thickness) of a deck of cards

- 1 cup egg substitute, such as Egg Beaters, or 6 egg whites, both of which can be cooked quickly in a microwave

Acceptable: Consume at least 20 grams of high-quality protein—either from a whey-casein protein blend, 100 percent whey protein, or solid food—anywhere from 1 hour before to 1 hour after your workout. Then eat a regular meal (Fat-Burning Time Zone) within 2 hours after your training session.

THE MUSCLE-BUILDING TIME ZONE: PROTEIN + CARBOHYDRATES

THE IDEAL

• Prepare a protein shake (made with water or milk) that provides at least 40 grams of whey and for casein protein, and 40 to 80 grams of carbohydrates. When choosing a product, look for one that contains little or no fat. As for carbohydrates, this is the one time when sugar is perfectly acceptable. That's because it can be used immediately for energy during your workout, and provides an insulin spike to slow protein breakdown—speeding muscle growth—after your workout. It's okay if you overshoot on the protein, but put a cap on your carb intake at the recommended 80 grams. Three products that fit our criteria:

- Biotest Surge Recovery (1½ servings)

  Available at: www.t-nation.com

  Per serving (prepared with water): 25 grams protein, 46 grams carbohydrate, 2½ grams fat

- At Large Nutrition Opticen (1½ servings)

  Available at: www.atlargenutrition.com

  Per serving (prepared with water): 52 grams protein, 25 grams carbohydrate, 1.7 grams fat

- MET-Rx Xtreme Size Up (1 serving)

  Available at: www.metrx.com

  Per serving (prepared with water): 59 grams protein, 80 grams carbohydrate, 6 grams fat

• Drink half of the beverage 30 minutes before your workout; drink the other half immediately after your workout.

• Eat a Fat-Burning Time Zone meal or snack that contains high-quality protein within 30 minutes to 1 hour after your training session. (Keep in mind, your Fat-Burning Time Zone snack could be another 20- to 40-gram protein shake, made without the carbs.)

PRACTICAL ALTERNATIVES

Good: Consume at least 20 grams of high-quality protein and 40 grams of carbohydrates, in the form of solid food or milk, 1 hour before your workout. Then eat a Fat-Burning Time Zone meal within an hour after your training session ends.

To accomplish the first task, you'll need to do a bit of mixing and matching. For instance, a turkey sandwich will do nicely here. Each slice of bread has 15 to 20 grams of carbohydrates—for a total of about 40 grams—and 4 slices of turkey has in the neighborhood of 20 grams of protein. Because vegetables contain very few carbs, include as many of them as desired, along with fat-free condiments such as mustard and horseradish. For simplicity, we've created a short list of protein and carbohydrate foods that you can easily combine to satisfy these guidelines (see opposite page). But in a pinch, just opt for a 16-ounce carton of low-fat chocolate milk. It provides about 16 grams of protein and 50 grams of carbohydrates—which is close enough on both counts. Or even better, check out the health food section of your grocery store for low-fat, fruit-flavored kefir (see page 60 for a description), which provides 28 grams of protein and 50 grams of carbs in every 16 ounces.

From Meat to Muscle

How steak makes it to your biceps:

1. The process starts in your mouth with the mechanical digestion of food: Your teeth cut, tear, and pulverize the steak into smaller particles, mixing it with saliva, to form a semisolid lump.

2. Once swallowed, the pulverized beef moves down the esophagus and empties into your stomach. Here, enzymes such as pepsin chemically break the steak into strands of amino acids. The whole mess is now more of a liquid, called *chyme.*

3. From the stomach, the chyme passes into the small intestines. Here additional enzymes—trypsin and chymotrypsin—act on the amino acid strands to break them into even smaller parts, until only single and double amino acids remain.

4. The amino acids are then transported through the cells that line the wall of the intestines and reach the bloodstream, in a process called *absorption.* They're now ready to be sent to your muscles via your blood vessels.

5. Once in the bloodstream, the amino acids are delivered directly to the muscle fibers via capillaries. There they aid in the repair of damaged muscle tissue. In fact, muscle protein synthesis can't occur unless amino acids are readily available—all the more reason to eat protein before you work out.

- Foods with 20 grams of protein:
  - 1 small can (3½ ounces) tuna
  - 3 to 4 ounces (3 to 4 slices) lean deli meat, such as turkey or chicken
  - 1 serving of any kind of lean meat that's about the size (length, width, and thickness) of a deck of cards
  - 1 cup egg substitute, such as Egg Beaters, or 6 egg whites, both of which can be cooked quickly in a microwave
- Foods with 15 to 20 grams of carbohydrates (you need a total of 2 servings):
  - 1 slice bread
  - ½ cup cooked pasta
  - ½ cup cooked rice
  - ½ cup cereal
  - ½ medium potato
  - 1 cup berries or sliced fruit
  - 1 whole apple, orange, or peach
  - ½ large banana
- Foods that contain both protein and carbohydrates (per 8-ounce cup):

FOOD	PROTEIN	CARBS
Milk	8 g	12 g
Chocolate milk	8 g	25 g
Plain yogurt	8 g	12 g
Fruit yogurt	8 g	25 g
Kefir	14 g	12 g
Flavored kefir	14 g	25 g
Cottage cheese	31 g	8 g

Acceptable: Consume at least 20 grams of high-quality protein and 40 grams of carbohydrates—from a protein shake, solid food, or milk—anywhere from 1 hour before to 1 hour after your workout. Then eat a Fat-Burning Time Zone meal within 2 hours after your training session.

What About Creatine?

We like it—and recommend it. Why? Because an unprecedented number of studies have shown that creatine supplementation is not only safe, but it also enhances both muscle size and strength gains when taken in conjunction with a resistance-training program.

How it works: Creatine helps speed your body's production of phosphocreatine, a high-energy compound in your muscles. The upshot is that this gives your body more of the fuel that's needed to lift heavy weights. For example, in one study, researchers found that guys who were given creatine were able to perform 12 repetitions with a weight that they could only complete 10 repetitions with before they started taking the supplement. In fact, they completed a total of 8 repetitions more over 5 sets. That means they were able to do more work and challenge their muscles harder, a benefit that translates into better gains. Case in point: In a recent paper, we reviewed dozens of studies and determined that creatine supplementation plus weight training, on average, results in about 5 pounds of additional muscle over a 12-week period. It's important to point out, though, that individual results will vary. People who have low muscle creatine levels tend to have the largest increases in muscle creatine after supplementation, and this translates into better gains in performance.

What to take: For best results, look for products that state "100% pure creatine monohydrate" on the label. (We like ProSource Creatine, available at www.prosource.net.)

Directions: Take 5 grams of creatine, mixed in water or a protein shake, four times a day for 7 days. This is called "loading," and although some experts don't think it's necessary, we've seen it to be an effective way to quickly saturate your muscles with creatine. After day 7, take 5 grams of creatine in the Muscle-Building Time Zone (before your workout is optimal), as well as anytime you want on the days you don't exercise.

PART III: FUEL

CHAPTER 8

THE DRINK LIST

Remember these seven words: Stick with beverages that contain no calories. For the most part, that means water, coffee, tea, and diet soda. These are your choices because most drinks—other than those already mentioned—are packed with carbohydrates, which are off-limits during the Fat-Burning Time Zone.

In addition, liquid calories are far easier to overconsume than those in solid food. They also tend to have little impact on appetite. For instance, in a recent study, Pennsylvania State University researchers fed men lunch once a week for 6 weeks, along with either a 12- or 18-ounce regular soda, diet soda, or water. The result: The study participants ate the same amount of food no matter the size or type of beverage served. Which means the men consumed significantly fewer total calories when they drank water or diet soda compared with the calorie-packed regular soda. What's more, their ratings of satiety and hunger were identical after each lunch, showing that the extra calories provided by the regular pop had no benefit.

So skip the caloric drinks and focus on beverages for hydration. And don't forget the other valuable compounds—such as antioxidants—that some of the beverages for hydration provide. Keep in mind that this guideline doesn't apply to protein shakes. Because unlike other beverages, protein shakes are filling and have been shown to reduce appetite. Also, since carbohydrates are encouraged in the Reloading Time Zone, you can add milk, kefir, and 100 percent fruit and vegetable juices to your drink list at that time. As for alcohol, we like it and, in fact, think it's perfectly fine to drink in moderation. It does have its downsides, though, which we'll explain in the pages that follow.

In short, simply drink as many no-calorie beverages—water, coffee, tea, and diet drinks—as you desire, and you may allow yourself as many as one or two alcoholic beverages per day. For more details on each type of beverage, read on.

TNT-Approved Beverages

Water

Coffee

Any type of unsweetened tea

No-calorie beverages

Alcohol, in moderation

WATER

As a general rule, try to drink 8 to 12 ounces of water for every 2 hours you're awake. That ensures that you're well hydrated, especially in the Fat-Burning Time Zone, since low-carbohydrate diets have a natural diuretic effect. This natural diuretic effect isn't bad; it just means your body isn't retaining as much water as normal and that you need to make sure you're providing it with plenty of incoming H_2O. Keep in mind that this is especially true if you drink caffeinated beverages—coffee, tea, diet soda—which also act as diuretics.

Why is proper hydration so important? For starters, researchers at Loma Linda University found that guys who drank five 8-ounce glasses of water a day were 54 percent less likely to suffer a fatal heart attack than those who drank two or fewer. But it's also critical for your muscles. That's because they're composed of about 80 percent water. Consequently, even as little as a 1 percent decrease in body water has been shown to impair exercise performance and adversely affect recovery. Not only that, but adequate water intake also helps you build muscle faster. Researchers in Germany found that protein synthesis occurs at a higher rate in muscle cells that are well hydrated. The bottom line: Water is good; drink lots of it.

COFFEE

If you rely on a couple of cups of coffee to jump-start your morning, here's good news: After years of research, most health experts regard it as not only safe, but highly recommended. In fact, a recent study in the *Journal of the American Medical Association* found no evidence of an association between heart disease risk and coffee consumption of up to six cups per day. Plus, it's packed with disease-fighting antioxidants. In the Fat-Burning Time Zone, use cream to flavor; in the Reloading Time Zone, use milk. In any time zone, you can use products such as NutraSweet, Equal, Splenda, or Sweet'N Low to sweeten. The best choice at Starbucks? A Caffè Americano, which is nearly carb-free: A 16-ounce grande contains just 3 grams of carbs, an amount not even worth worrying about it.

TEA

Tea is widely known for its beneficial health effects. And you can thank its high content of catechins—antioxidants that help fight cancer, heart disease, and Alzheimer's. Tea also helps reduce stress, according to researchers in the United Kingdom. In the study, men drank either four cups of black tea daily, or a placebo beverage that contained the same amount of caffeine. After 6 weeks, the study participants were then asked to engage in stressful activities while scientists monitored their physiological and psychological anxiety. The result? The tea drinkers exhibited 20 percent lower levels of stress hormones than those who drank the faux tea. They also reported *feeling* more relaxed than did the placebo group. The likely reason: Antioxidants in the tea may act on areas of your brain that calm your central nervous system.

How to Wake Up Your Brain

If you're feeling drowsy at work, don't be tempted to reach for a soda. British researchers discovered that people who downed a sugary drink containing 42 milligrams of sugar and 30 milligrams of caffeine—the amount in a 12-ounce cola—exhibited slower reaction times and a greater number of lapses in attention for the next 90 minutes compared with those who sipped a sugar-free beverage. Although a sugar rush has been shown to boost cognitive performance, the effect is short-lived, lasting just 10 to 15 minutes.

Your best option for a brain boost: a sugar-free drink, such as 8 ounces of black, unsweetened coffee that delivers 100 milligrams of caffeine. When Austrian scientists measured brain activity in 15 men after they consumed either 100 milligrams of caffeine—about the same amount as in a cup of joe—or a placebo, test results showed that the caffeine drinkers registered higher levels of activity in the regions of the brain responsible for short-term memory, attention, and concentration. Although researchers aren't sure why caffeine boosts brainpower, they speculate that it may improve cerebral blood flow and the transmission of nerve signals. However, there's a time limit for coffee, too: In the study, the benefits diminished after 45 minutes, but without the brain crash that occurs with sugar drinks.

Although green tea gets the most press, black and herbal teas provide similar health benefits. To get the most from any product, steep your tea for at least 3 minutes; any less than that results in lower amounts of the disease-fighting antioxidants. Just as with coffee, you can flavor with cream (Fat-Burning Time Zone) or milk (Reloading Time Zone) and use artificial sweeteners as desired.

DIET BEVERAGES

Diet sodas and other diet drinks such as Crystal Light make our list for one reason: They have 5 or fewer calories per serving. (That's a negligible amount.) As a result, these beverages have no physiological effect on your ability to lose fat. However, they also don't have any health benefits to tout. So feel free to drink them, but in addition to the recommended amount of water, and with the knowledge that unsweetened coffee and tea are better choices.

Also, a quick word about artificial sweeteners: The majority of research on aspartame (NutraSweet), sucralose (Splenda), and saccharin (Sweet'N Low) shows them to be safe for human consumption. Yet there are some rodent studies, as well as anecdotal reports in humans, that suggest they may carry negative side effects in high amounts. What's that mean to you? Don't consume them in huge amounts! We can't say that doing so would cause you any health problems, but it does lead to one problem: You drink less of everything else. For instance, one or two diet sodas a day is fine, but if you're downing five or six 12-ounce bottles, then that means you're limiting your intake of healthful beverages, particularly water.

Rooibos: The Naturally Sweet Tea

Rooibos (ROY-bus) is a vibrant red tea made from a South African legume. The tea is caffeine free and also naturally sweet, so you won't need to add sugar.

Why it's healthy: Rooibos is loaded with disease-fighting antioxidants. Pakistani researchers found that it lowers blood pressure in rodents. It's also been shown to boost the immune system—in fact, a recent Japanese study on mice and rats suggests that rooibos tea may help prevent allergies and even cancer.

Where to find it: Look for Celestial Seasonings rooibos teas (we like Madagascar Vanilla Red) in your local grocery store, or try one from Adagio, an organic product that features 13 different all-natural flavors (www.adagio.com).

ALCOHOL

When it comes to alcohol we think the phrase, "you can get too much of a good thing" is right on the money, but not because of a bad frat-party experience. In moderation, alcohol appears to improve levels of good cholesterol and has a relaxing, stress-reducing effect. Plus, you might not realize it, but

---

The Missing Ingredient

There's one key figure you won't find listed on a nutrition label: caffeine content. So, to determine how much of a jolt you can expect from popular diet soft drinks, University of Florida researchers decided to analyze them. Below, we've highlighted the diet beverages tested, and compared them with the gold standard—a regular black coffee from Dunkin' Donuts.

Dunkin' Donuts Regular Coffee
143 milligrams per 16 ounces, **8.9 milligrams** per ounce

Red Bull Sugarfree
64.7 milligrams per 8.3 ounces, **7.8 milligrams** per ounce

Diet Coke with Lime
39.6 milligrams per 12 ounces, **3.3 milligrams** per ounce

Diet Coke
38.2 milligrams per 12 ounces, **3.2 milligrams** per ounce

Diet Dr Pepper
33.8 milligrams per 12 ounces, **2.8 milligrams** per ounce

Diet Pepsi
27.4 milligrams per 12 ounces, **2.3 milligrams** per ounce

Diet 7-Up, Sprite, and Caffeine-Free Diet Coke
zero milligram per 12 ounces, **zero milligram** per ounce

wine and hard liquor don't contain carbohydrates, and "light" beers only have a couple of grams of carbs per 12-ounce serving.

The downside is that excessive amounts of alcohol prevent your body from burning fat for energy. This effect is exacerbated when combined with carbohydrates, such as those found in regular beer or in mixers. (See "How Alcohol Makes You Fat," page 94.) So it's important not to overdo it. You

---

Avoid a Killer Hangover

Binge drinking can literally lead to a killer hangover. Harvard University researchers found that throwing back a few too many alcoholic beverages can elevate a person's risk of atrial fibrillation—a condition that may up your stroke risk by 500 percent. Your safe limit? Three drinks in a 24-hour period, says study author Kenneth Mukamal, MD. Trouble is, a new report from Duke University shows that the Harvard study's definition of a standard drink differs substantially from the amount an average guy is apt to pour for himself. Here's how the two compare, drink by drink.

Wine

The Harvard standard: 4 ounces
The average guy's: 7 ounces

Beer

The Harvard standard: 12 ounces
The average guy's: 13 ounces

Shot

The Harvard standard: 1.25 ounces
The average guy's: 2 ounces

Mixed Drink

The Harvard standard: 1.25 ounces*
The average guy's: 4.2 ounces*

* Denotes amount of liquor

can toe the line by sticking with one or two drinks—at most—per day. In fact, you'll find a glass of wine makes the perfect complement to any meal. (It's also great as a "dessert.")

THE RULES FOR BELLYING UP TO THE BAR

1. Avoid mixing alcohol with any type of fruit juice or non-diet soda, which add unnecessary calories and carbohydrates. Combined with alcohol, these can lead to fat storage.

2. Avoid regular beer. It's packed with carbohydrates. Go with a light beer that contains less than 3 grams carbohydrates per 12-ounce serving.

TNT-APPROVED ALCOHOL	
TYPE OF ALCOHOL	ONE DRINK
Wine	4 oz
Light beer	12 oz
Gin	1¼ oz
Rum	1¼ oz
Whiskey	1¼ oz
Vodka	1¼ oz

Broaden Your Wine List

Red or white? Just say yes, according to a new study from the University of Connecticut. Although previous research only touted the cardiovascular benefits of drinking red varietals, scientists discovered that white wine may protect your heart just as well as cabernet and merlot. To make the white variety, winemakers remove the grapes' skins—which give red wine its color—before fermentation. Because the skin is the only part of the grape that contains resveratrol, an antioxidant that improves blood flow to the heart, it was assumed that red was far more healthy. Not so, says study author Dipak K. Das, PhD, whose laboratory determined that an unidentified antioxidant in white wine offers similar heart protection. The bottom line: "Consumption of one to two glasses of either red or white wine daily should be equally beneficial," says Dr. Das.

How Alcohol Makes You Fat

1. You take a swig of beer, a sip of wine, or a shot of vodka.

2. Within seconds, the beverage passes through your esophagus into your stomach.

3. From your stomach, 20 percent of the alcohol is absorbed immediately into your bloodstream; the rest moves on to your intestines and is absorbed from there.

4. Once in your bloodstream, the alcohol travels directly to your liver, where it's immediately broken down (because it's toxic to the body). During this process, waste products called acetate and acetaldehyde are created.

5. Acetate and acetaldehyde signal your body to stop burning fat. What's more, your body also starts manufacturing fat from another waste product of alcohol, acetyl CoA.

6. Your body can effectively process only 0.5 to 1 ounce of alcohol per hour. However, the more you drink, the longer your body is inhibited from burning fat, and the more fat that builds up from all the excess acetyl CoA. (A 12-ounce beer contains about 0.6 ounce of alcohol.)

7. If you drink an alcoholic beverage that's also high in carbohydrates—such as regular beer or a cocktail mixed with fruit juice—you'll further promote fat gain, because the carbohydrates will raise your levels of insulin, a hormone that triggers your body to store fat.

CHAPTER 9

RECIPES FOR SUCCESS

O ver the years, one of the most important things we've learned is that no one really likes "diet food." It's typically thought of as bland, and conjures images of plain grilled chicken breasts and run-of-the-mill salads. This, of course, is a major flaw in any eating plan that you want people to stick with. Food plays a big part in our culture, so removing the pleasure from it leaves you feeling that you're missing out on one of life's great experiences. Which is why we believe that food, and particularly "diet food," should be thoroughly enjoyed. Savored, even.

Thankfully, this isn't a problem with the foods that are allowed on the TNT Diet. Of course, creating delicious meals does take a bit of effort and know-how. However, if you can spare 15 to 30 minutes for the former, we've supplied the latter, with the recipes that follow. They're what we describe as "simple, but sophisticated." That's because while easy to make, these dishes are also packed with bold flavors that will please even the most discerning palate. The best part is that by always making a little extra, your taste buds can enjoy an encore performance at the next day's lunch. All of which will help you stick with your eating plan because you *want* to—not because you have to. And that's ultimately the best recipe for success.

For each recipe, we've indicated whether it's intended for the Fat-Burning Time Zone or the Reloading Time Zone, or in a few cases, both. Note that some recipes are full meals—for instance, both a meat and vegetable dish—and others are just one or the other. Consider the full meals merely suggestions, and feel free to mix and match any of the dishes as you desire, as long as they fit into the same Time Zone.

As for amounts, let your appetite dictate how much you eat. You'll notice that we haven't provided servings or calorie counts for any of the meals. This is intentional, since the TNT Diet will automatically regulate your intake. For reference, though, you'll find that the recipes each make about three to four conventional servings—typically perfect for a couple. So if you're a single guy, you may want to cut the recipes in half, and if you're cooking for a family, you might want to double them.

Also, keep in mind that although dried spices and herbs are often suggested in the recipes, this is just for convenience. Anytime you have the fresh stuff available, we highly recommend it.

Ready to get cookin'? *Bon appétit.*

Fat-Burning Time Zone

NEXGEN MUFFINS

This ready-to-eat muffin, created by our friend Keith Berkowitz, MD, contains 10 grams of high-quality protein, no sugar, and 24 grams of fiber. Remember, although fiber is a carbohydrate, it's nondigestible, so in effect, it doesn't count. That makes these muffins a great Fat-Burning Time Zone alternative to eating scrambled eggs or omelets. How do they do it? Instead of using wheat flour, Dr. Berkowitz and his team substitute a blend of six natural fibers that have been ground into a fine powder. And since eggs provide the protein, each muffin contains all of the essential nutrients that your muscles need for growth. They're available in Lemon Poppy Seed, Banana Walnut, and Orange Pineapple at www.nexgenfoods.com.

Fat-Burning Time Zone

HALLOUMI CHEESE

When Mary Dan Eades, MD, coauthor of *Protein Power,* told us about a Greek cheese that made a great substitute for toast and pancakes, we had our doubts. But then we tried it for ourselves. And sure enough, it doesn't melt when you grill it—it simply browns like a pancake. (Just add sugar-free syrup.) It's packed with protein and contains almost no carbohydrates. Look for it in the specialty cheese section of grocery stores, or online at www.halloumicheese.com.

Fat-Burning Time Zone

CREAM CAKES

⅔ cup cream
6 eggs, beaten
Olive oil
Butter or sugar-free syrup

1. Whisk the cream into the beaten eggs until the mixture is well combined. Heat about 2 tablespoons olive oil in a nonstick omelet skillet over medium-high heat. Slowly pour in some of the egg mixture until it covers the surface (it should look like a thin pancake). Let cook until the surface is just set. Flip the cream cake, and cook for 30 to 60 seconds longer. Remove from the heat.

2. Repeat to make 5 or 6 cakes. Top with butter or sugar-free syrup for a low-carb pancake.

Fat-Burning Time Zone

STEAK SALAD

To make this into a Reloading Time Zone meal, serve with a baked sweet potato or any other nutrient-dense carb of your choice.

Marinade and Steak

¼   cup olive oil
     Juice of ½ lemon
2   teaspoons Dijon mustard
1   teaspoon dried oregano
1   teaspoon dried basil
1   teaspoon chopped garlic
     Salt and freshly ground pepper
1   flank steak (1½ to 2 pounds)

Salad

½   cup pine nuts
1   head Boston or Bibb lettuce, torn into bite-size pieces
1   bunch frisée, torn into bite-size pieces
1   pint grape tomatoes
2   jarred roasted red peppers, sliced
1   package (4 ounces) crumbled blue cheese

Dressing

⅔   cup olive oil
½   cup white balsamic vinegar (or red wine vinegar)
1   tablespoon Dijon mustard
     Salt and freshly ground pepper

1. For the steak: Combine the olive oil, lemon juice, mustard, oregano, basil, garlic, and salt and pepper in a small bowl. In a large bowl, pour the marinade over the beef; marinate for 20 to 30 minutes.

2. Heat a grill or grill pan over medium-high heat. Grill the steak 8 to 10 minutes on each side or to desired doneness. Let rest for 5 to 10 minutes. Cut into thin slices.

3. Meanwhile, make the salad and dressing: Place the pine nuts in a small sauté pan and heat to medium-high. Cook, tossing frequently, until evenly browned, being careful not to burn.

4. In a large salad bowl, combine the lettuce, frisée, tomatoes, red pepper slices, cheese, and toasted pine nuts and toss.

5. In a small bowl, combine the olive oil, vinegar, mustard, and salt and pepper and whisk well.

6. Divide the salad among dinner plates, place the sliced beef on top, and drizzle with the dressing.

Fat-Burning Time Zone

TACO SALAD

To make this into a Reloading Time Zone meal, serve with whole wheat tortillas or any other nutrient-dense carb of your choice.

1 pound ground beef
1 package taco seasoning, plus water as directed on the package
2 cups red bell pepper strips
¼ cup salsa of your choice, plus more for serving
8 cups shredded romaine lettuce
2 cups diced tomatoes
2 cups shredded pepper jack cheese
1 cup sour cream

1. Cook the ground beef in a large skillet over medium heat until browned. Add the taco seasoning and water, peppers, and ¼ cup salsa and simmer until the vegetables are al dente.

2. Arrange the lettuce and tomatoes on salad plates and spoon the taco mixture on top. Serve with shredded cheese, sour cream, and additional salsa.

A sliced avocado is a great addition to this salad.

Fat-Burning Time Zone

TUNA SALAD

To make this a Reloading Time Zone meal, spread the salad on 2 slices of 100 percent whole wheat bread for a Tuna Salad Sandwich.

2	cans (6 ounces each) white albacore tuna packed in water
1	red bell pepper, chopped into small pieces
1	stalk celery, diced
¾	cup mayonnaise
1	dill pickle, diced
1	tablespoon capers, plus a sprinkling of the brine they're packed in
2	teaspoons Dijon mustard
½	teaspoon dried dill weed
	Freshly ground black pepper to taste
6	leaves of romaine lettuce heart (see note)

1. Mix the tuna, bell pepper, celery, mayonnaise, pickle, capers and a sprinkle of their brine, mustard, dill, and black pepper in a bowl.

2. Arrange the romaine leaves on plates. Spoon the salad into the leaves, leaving enough room to fold the lettuce over.

Note: For a different taste, use Belgian endive or radicchio instead of the romaine.

Fat-Burning Time Zone

ALMOND-CRUSTED CHICKEN

To make this a Reloading Time Zone Meal, substitute 100 percent whole wheat flour for the ground almonds to enjoy Breaded Chicken.

    1   package (6 ounces) slivered almonds
    ½   cup grated Parmesan cheese
    1   teaspoon dried rosemary
    1   teaspoon dried basil
        Salt and freshly ground pepper to taste
    2   eggs
    1½ pounds boneless chicken breasts (3 or 4 breasts)
    2   tablespoons olive oil

1. Preheat the oven to 385°F. Line a baking sheet with foil.

2. In a food processor, grind the almonds to the consistency of bread crumbs. In a shallow bowl, combine the almonds, cheese, rosemary, basil, salt, and pepper. In another shallow bowl, gently whisk the eggs until combined. In an assembly line, dip each chicken breast in the egg, then coat with the nut mixture (see note).

3. Heat the olive oil in a large nonstick sauté pan over medium–high heat. Add the chicken and cook each side for 4 to 5 minutes, or until the almond coating starts to brown. Add more oil if the pan begins to appear dry.

4. Place the chicken on the prepared baking sheet and bake for 20 to 30 minutes, until golden brown and cooked through.

Note: If you have time, refrigerate the chicken for 10 to 15 minutes after you've dipped it into the egg and ground almonds. It will help the coating stick during cooking.

Fat-Burning Time Zone

GREEN BEANS WITH TOASTED PINE NUTS

1   pound fresh green beans
¼   cup pine nuts
3   tablespoons olive oil
     Salt and freshly ground pepper to taste

1. In a large sauté pan, bring 5 cups water to a boil. Drop the green beans into the water and cook for 3 to 4 minutes. Drain in a colander, then run cold water over them for a few seconds to stop the cooking process. This will ensure that you don't end up with soft and mushy beans.

2. In the same pan, cook the pine nuts in 1 tablespoon of the olive oil over medium heat, stirring, until the nuts begin to turn golden brown. Return the green beans to the pan along with the remaining 2 tablespoons of olive oil and salt and pepper to taste. Sauté until the beans are heated through.

Fat-Burning Time Zone

CHICKEN CURRY

1–1½   pounds boneless chicken breasts, cut into 1-inch cubes
     Salt and freshly ground pepper
2   tablespoons olive oil
1   can (14½ ounces) diced tomatoes
1   cup chicken broth
½   cup white wine
1   heaping tablespoon curry powder
½   cup cream

1. Season the chicken with salt and pepper. Heat the olive oil over medium-high heat in a large sauté pan. Add the chicken and cook, stirring, until no longer pink.

2. Add the tomatoes, broth, wine, and curry powder, and bring to a boil. Reduce the heat, cover, and simmer for 20 to 25 minutes, until the mixture has reduced by half. Add the cream and simmer for 5 minutes longer, until the curry thickens.

Fat-Burning Time Zone and Reloading Time Zone

ROASTED BROCCOLI

2 broccoli crowns
3 tablespoons olive oil
   Salt and freshly ground pepper

1. Preheat the oven to 385°F.

2. Trim the broccoli into bite-size florets. Place on a baking sheet. Pour the olive oil over the broccoli and season with salt and pepper. Using your hands, toss, making sure each floret is covered with oil.

3. Roast for 15 to 20 minutes, tossing with a spatula once or twice, until the florets begin to brown.

Fat-Burning Time Zone

CHICKEN STIR-FRY

To make this into a Reloading Time Zone meal, serve over brown rice or with any other nutrient-dense carb of your choice.

4	tablespoons olive oil (see note)
1–1½	pounds boneless chicken breasts, cut into strips
1	cup chicken broth
3	tablespoons Thai peanut sauce
2	tablespoons soy sauce
½	teaspoon chopped garlic
½	teaspoon ground ginger
1	red bell pepper, cut into strips
1	orange bell pepper, cut into strips
1	package (8 to 10 ounces) mushrooms (any variety), sliced
1	cup snow peas
1	cup cashews

1. In a large sauté pan, heat 1 tablespoon of the olive oil over medium–high heat. Add the chicken strips and sauté until no longer pink. Add the broth, peanut sauce, soy sauce, garlic, and ginger. Simmer for about 20 minutes.

2. When the chicken has almost finished cooking, sauté the peppers and mushrooms with 2 tablespoons olive oil in a separate pan for 4 to 5 minutes. If you like, add a tablespoon of sauce from the chicken.

3. Add the snow peas to the vegetables and cook for 2 minutes. Combine the chicken and vegetables and remove from heat.

4. In an empty sauté pan, sauté the cashews in the remaining 1 tablespoon olive oil until they begin to brown. Sprinkle on top of the chicken and veggies and serve.

Note: In place of olive oil, you can also use the same amount of Drew's Thai Sesame Lime dressing (www.chefdrew.com).

Don't add the nuts to the stir-fry until you're ready to eat—they'll get soggy.

Fat-Burning Time Zone

CHICKEN WITH PANCETTA AND ASIAGO

1–1½ pounds boneless chicken breasts (3 to 4 breasts)
  ½ cup jarred pesto
  2 tablespoons olive oil
  4 ounces sliced pancetta, cut into small squares (see note)
  1 can (14½ ounces) diced tomatoes
  1 can (8 ounces) tomato sauce
  1 teaspoon dried rosemary
  1 teaspoon dried basil
  1 teaspoon dried oregano
  4 thin slices Asiago cheese

1. Slather the chicken with the pesto. Heat the olive oil over medium–high heat in a large nonstick pan. Add the chicken and sear for 4 minutes per side. Remove the chicken from the pan and set aside.

2. Add the pancetta to the pan and sauté until crispy. Add the tomatoes, tomato sauce, rosemary, basil, and oregano and stir. Return the chicken to the sauce and simmer for 20 to 30 minutes, or until cooked through and no longer pink.

3. Place the cheese on top of each breast, cover, and cook a few minutes more, until the cheese is melted.

Note: You can usually find sliced pancetta prepackaged in your grocery store's deli. It's delicious as an addition to any Italian dish or just as a snack.

Fat-Burning Time Zone
and Reloading Time Zone

ROASTED ZUCCHINI

2 zucchini
2 tablespoons olive oil
  Salt and freshly ground black pepper (see note)

Preheat the oven to 400°F. Slice the zucchini into 1-inch-thick coins. Place on a baking sheet and coat with the olive oil, salt, and pepper. Roast for 10 minutes, until al dente.

Note: We also love to use Nando's Peri-Peri grinds (www.nandosusa.com) for added flavor.

Fat-Burning Time Zone

ROASTED CHICKEN

To make this into a Reloading Time Zone meal, serve with a baked sweet potato or any other nutrient-dense carb of your choice.

 1 fryer chicken (3 to 4 pounds), giblets removed
 ½ lemon
 3 tablespoons olive oil
 1 teaspoon dried rosemary
 1 teaspoon dried basil
 1 teaspoon dried oregano
 1 teaspoon dried parsley
    Salt and freshly ground pepper

1. Preheat the oven to 425°F. Rinse the chicken inside and out and pat dry.

2. Squeeze the juice from the lemon half into a small bowl; set aside the squeezed half. Stir the olive oil, rosemary, basil, oregano, and parsley into the lemon juice in the bowl. Rub the mixture over the chicken and season with salt and pepper. Place the lemon half in the cavity.

3. Place the chicken in a roasting pan and roast for 45 minutes to 1 hour, until the skin is nicely browned and an instant-read thermometer inserted in the thickest part of a thigh registers 165°F.

This is where fresh herbs come in handy. If you have them, place several sprigs inside the chicken with the lemon. It adds to the flavor during roasting.

Fat-Burning Time Zone and Reloading Time Zone

ROASTED BUTTERNUT SQUASH AND ONIONS

1 large butternut squash, rind removed, and chopped into chunks
1 large Mayan sweet onion, quartered
2 tablespoons olive oil
  Juice of ½ lemon
  Salt and freshly ground pepper

1. When there are about 15 or 20 minutes remaining to roast the chicken (Roasted Chicken, page 108), scatter the squash and the onion quarters in the pan around the chicken (see note). Drizzle with the olive oil and lemon juice and season with salt and pepper.

2. Continue roasting, tossing the vegetables with the pan drippings once or twice, for 20 minutes. The vegetables are done when the squash is fork tender and the onion begins to brown.

Note: If roasting the chicken on a rack, remove it when you add the vegetables and set the chicken directly on top of the vegetables. Otherwise, juices from the chicken won't come in contact with the squash and onion, which makes them tastier.

Reloading Time Zone

PENNE PUTTANESCA WITH CHICKEN

      2   tablespoons olive oil
1–1½   pounds boneless chicken breasts (3 to 4 breasts)
          Salt and freshly ground pepper
      1   cup red wine
      1   can (14½ ounces) diced tomatoes
      1   can (8 ounces) tomato sauce
      1   cup kalamata olives
      1   tablespoon capers
      1   teaspoon dried oregano
      1   teaspoon dried basil
      1   pound whole wheat penne (or any whole wheat, bite-size pasta)

1. In a large sauté pan, heat the olive oil over medium-high heat. Season the chicken with salt and pepper and add to pan. Sear 4 to 5 minutes per side, until chicken is cooked through and beginning to brown.

2. Remove the chicken from pan and set aside. While the pan is still hot, add the wine and stir. When the wine begins to simmer, add the tomatoes, tomato sauce, olives, capers, oregano, and basil.

3. Slice the chicken into small strips and add to the sauce. Simmer for at least 30 minutes.

4. Meanwhile, cook the pasta in a large pot of boiling water according to package directions. Serve with the chicken and sauce.

Fat-Burning Time Zone

BRATS AND SAUERKRAUT

2   tablespoons olive oil
1   pound bratwurst
1   bag (2 pounds) fresh sauerkraut (or you can use the canned variety)
    Freshly ground black pepper

1. Preheat the oven to 350°F.

2. In a large sauté pan coated with olive oil, cook the bratwursts over medium heat until they begin to brown on all sides.

3. Drain some of the liquid from the sauerkraut and discard. Place the sauerkraut in an 8-inch-square baking dish. Season with pepper and stir.

4. Arrange the brats on top of the sauerkraut. Bake for 15 to 20 minutes, until the sauerkraut is bubbly and the brats are cooked through.

Fat-Burning Time Zone and Reloading Time Zone

SAUTÉED BRUSSELS SPROUTS

1½ pounds brussels sprouts
2   tablespoons olive oil
    Salt and freshly ground pepper
1   cup white wine

1. Clean the brussels sprouts by removing the outer layer of leaves (including any visible blemishes) and trimming the stems.

2. Heat the olive oil over medium–high heat in a large nonstick pan. Add the sprouts and season with salt and pepper. Cook for 2 to 3 minutes, until the oil is absorbed. Add ¼ cup of the wine and stir. As the wine cooks off, the sprouts will begin to brown. Cook for about 5 minutes, stirring occasionally, until all of the moisture has been absorbed. Add the remaining ¾ cup wine and continue to cook, stirring, 6 to 10 minutes, or until the sprouts are nicely browned and al dente. Don't worry about burning the brussels sprouts a bit; the toasty color really adds flavor to this dish.

Fat-Burning Time Zone

ROSEMARY PORK TENDERLOIN

To make this into a Reloading Time Zone meal, serve with brown rice or any other nutrient-dense carb of your choice.

- 1 pork tenderloin
- 2 tablespoons olive oil
- 2 teaspoons Dijon mustard
- 1 teaspoon chopped garlic
- 1 tablespoon dried rosemary
- 1 teaspoon dried oregano
  Salt and freshly ground pepper to taste

1. Preheat the oven to 375°F.

2. Place the tenderloin in a rectangular baking dish. Combine the olive oil, mustard, garlic, rosemary, oregano, salt, and pepper in a small bowl. Slather the mixture on the pork using your hands or a basting brush.

3. Bake the tenderloin, uncovered, for 40 to 45 minutes, until the pork is no longer pink in the center. Cut into 1-inch slices to serve.

Fat-Burning Time Zone

MASHED CAULIFLOWER

- 1 head cauliflower, cut into bite-size pieces
- ½ cup chicken broth
- ½ cup sour cream
- 1 tablespoon butter
  Salt and freshly ground pepper

1. Bring a large pot of water to a boil. Add the cauliflower and boil until fork tender, about 10 minutes; drain.

2. Combine the cauliflower in a large mixing bowl with the broth, sour cream, and butter. With an electric mixer, beat on high until smooth. Season with salt and pepper.

Fat-Burning Time Zone

SAUSAGE WITH FETA AND SPINACH

To make this into a Reloading Time Zone meal, prepare your favorite pasta—for instance, penne or ziti—and combine with other ingredients in Step 3. Bake as directed.

2	tablespoons olive oil
1–1½	pounds hot Italian sausage, cut into 1-inch-thick slices
1	can (14½ ounces) diced tomatoes
1	can (8 ounces) tomato sauce (see note)
1	teaspoon dried basil
1	teaspoon dried oregano
6	ounces crumbled plain feta cheese
1	bag (10 ounces) fresh spinach

1. Preheat the oven to 375°F.

2. Heat the olive oil over medium heat in large nonstick sauté pan. Add the sausage and cook, stirring, until browned and cooked through. Add the tomatoes, tomato sauce, basil, and oregano. Stir to combine.

3. Pour the mixture into a 3- to 4-quart casserole dish. Add the feta and spinach, stirring until all of the spinach is incorporated. Bake for 20 to 25 minutes, until bubbly.

Note: We've found that Contadina tomato sauce has less sugar than several other brands.

Reloading Time Zone

KIELBASA AND LENTIL SOUP

2 tablespoons olive oil
1 pound kielbasa
4 celery stalks, diced
2 carrots, diced
2 cups chicken broth
1 can (14½ ounces) diced tomatoes
½ cup dry lentils
1 bay leaf
1 turnip, chopped into 1-inch pieces
1 cup white button mushrooms, halved
Freshly ground pepper

1. Heat the olive oil over medium-high heat in a large pot. Add the kielbasa and sear on each side, 4 to 5 minutes. Transfer to a cutting board and cut into 1-inch pieces.

2. In the remaining oil in the pan, sauté the celery and carrots for 4 to 5 minutes. Add the broth, tomatoes, lentils, and bay leaf and simmer for 20 minutes. Add the kielbasa, turnip, and mushrooms and simmer for another 10 minutes, until the vegetables are tender. Discard the bay leaf. Season with pepper and serve.

Salt and other spices aren't necessary in this recipe. The flavorful kielbasa is enough to season the soup.

Reloading Time Zone

SAUSAGE AND RED PEPPER PIZZA

 1 unbaked prepared whole wheat pizza crust
 ½ jar pizza sauce (about 7 ounces)
 1 bag (8 ounces) shredded 2% mozzarella cheese
 8 ounces cooked turkey sausage or turkey pepperoni
 1 cup pitted black olives, chopped
 1 red bell pepper, thinly sliced
 1 teaspoon red pepper flakes

1. Preheat the oven according to pizza crust directions.

2. Spread the sauce over the crust, leaving a ½-inch border along the edge. Top with the cheese. Layer the rest of the toppings to your preference. You could use any other type of vegetable here—mushrooms, green peppers, and onions, to name a few.

3. Bake the pizza for 10 to 12 minutes, or until bubbly. Allow the pizza to rest for a minute or two before slicing.

Fat-Burning Time Zone

ASIAN STEAK STEW

1 flank or strip steak (1½ to 2 pounds)
2 tablespoons olive oil
1 cup water
1 cup chicken broth
½ cup white wine
2 tablespoons soy sauce
½ teaspoon ground ginger
2 cups snow peas
1 red bell pepper, sliced into thin strips
2 cups shredded cabbage (Savoy or Napa)

1. Cut the steak in half lengthwise and then slice into thin strips (see note). Heat the olive oil over medium-high heat in a large pot. Add the steak slices and cook until browned.

2. Add the water, broth, wine, and soy sauce. Bring to a simmer and cook for about 5 minutes. Stir in the ginger. Add the snow peas and red pepper, cover, and cook 5 minutes. Stir in the cabbage and simmer, stirring several times, until all of the vegetables are al dente, about 3 minutes.

Note: Cut the beef against the grain and the meat will be more tender.

Fat-Burning Time Zone

BEEF KEBABS

To make this into a Reloading Time Zone meal, serve with a baked sweet potato or any other nutrient-dense carb of your choice.

    1   red bell pepper, cut into large pieces
    1   orange bell pepper, cut into large pieces
    1   yellow bell pepper, cut into large pieces
    1   red onion, cut into large pieces
    1   package (8 to 10 ounces) mushrooms
    1   cup Italian dressing
  1½   pounds beef stew meat
        Metal or wooden skewers (see note)

1. Heat a grill or grill pan over medium-high heat.

2. Toss the peppers, onion, and mushrooms in a bowl with ½ cup of the dressing to evenly coat. In a separate bowl, combine the beef and remaining ½ cup dressing.

3. To have better control over varying cooking times, thread the beef and the vegetables onto separate skewers. Grill the vegetables until the edges of the peppers begin to blacken a bit. Grill the meat to desired doneness.

Note: Always soak wooden skewers in water first so they don't burn on the grill.

Fat-Burning Time Zone

CILANTRO FLANK STEAK

To make this into a Reloading Time Zone meal, serve with a baked sweet potato or any other nutrient-dense carb of your choice.

   Juice of ½ lime
2 tablespoons olive oil
1 tablespoon chopped fresh cilantro
1 teaspoon chopped garlic
1 flank steak (1½ to 2 pounds)
   Salt and freshly ground pepper

1. Heat a grill or grill pan over medium-high heat.

2. Combine the lime juice, olive oil, cilantro, and garlic in a small bowl. Slather the mixture on the steak and season with salt and pepper.

3. Place the steak on the grill and cook for 8 to 10 minutes each side or to desired doneness.

Fat-Burning Time Zone

AVOCADO AND TOMATO SALAD

To turn this into a Reloading Time Zone recipe, serve with sweet white corn.

    2   avocados, chopped into 1-inch pieces (see note)
    1   pint grape tomatoes, halved
        Juice of ½ lime
    1   teaspoon chopped fresh cilantro
        Salt and freshly ground pepper to taste
        Olive oil

Combine the avocados, tomatoes, lime juice, cilantro, and salt and pepper in a bowl. Drizzle with olive oil (about once around the bowl). Stir gently to combine.

Note: It's best to use firmer avocados in this recipe.

Fat-Burning Time Zone

CHILI

2	tablespoons olive oil
1	pound ground beef
1	red bell pepper, chopped
1	yellow bell pepper, chopped
1	teaspoon chopped garlic
1	can (14½ ounces) diced tomatoes
1	can (8 ounces) tomato sauce
½	cup water
2	tablespoons red wine vinegar
1	tablespoon Worcestershire sauce
¼	cup chili powder (or more, depending on the spice level you prefer)
1	tablespoon ground cumin
1	teaspoon ground coriander
½	teaspoon crushed red pepper flakes (or more, depending on your taste)
	Salt and freshly ground pepper
1	cup grated Cheddar or Monterey Jack cheese

1. Heat the olive oil in a large pot over medium heat. Add the ground beef and cook until browned.

2. Add the bell peppers, garlic, tomatoes, tomato sauce, water, vinegar, Worcestershire, chili powder, cumin, coriander, and pepper flakes and mix together. Cover and simmer, stirring occasionally for 20 to 30 minutes, until desired thickness. Taste, and season with salt and pepper. Serve with grated cheese sprinkled on top.

This recipe is delicious with a relish of chopped cherry tomatoes and pickles sprinkled on top.

Fat-Burning Time Zone

FILET MIGNON WITH TOMATO AND MOZZARELLA SALAD

Filet Mignon

4   beef tenderloins (filet mignon)
    Salt and freshly ground pepper

Salad

6   plum tomatoes, cut into bite-size segments
8   ounces fresh mozzarella cheese, cut into 1-inch cubes
    Salt and freshly ground pepper
    Olive oil
    Balsamic vinegar
    Fresh basil leaves

1. For the filet mignon: Heat a grill or grill pan over medium-high heat. Season the tenderloins with salt and pepper. Grill the tenderloins about 8 minutes each side, or until desired doneness.

2. For the salad: Combine the tomatoes and cheese in a bowl. Season with salt and pepper and toss gently. Drizzle generously with olive oil and vinegar (about twice around the bowl for each). Tear the basil leaves and sprinkle on top of the salad.

Fat-Burning Time Zone

MEATBALLS

To make this into a Reloading Time Zone meal, omit the cheese and serve the meatballs over pasta of your choice, such as spaghetti.

1½–2 pounds ground beef (85 percent lean, see note)
  1 egg
  ½ cup grated Parmesan cheese
  1 tablespoon low-carb ketchup
  2 teaspoons dried oregano
  1 teaspoon Worcestershire sauce
     Salt and freshly ground pepper
  2 tablespoons olive oil
  2 cans (8 ounces each) tomato sauce
  1 can (14½ ounces) diced tomatoes
  1 teaspoon dried basil
  1 teaspoon dried oregano
  8 ounces mozzarella cheese (fresh mozzarella is best), sliced

1. In a large bowl, combine the beef, egg, Parmesan, ketchup, oregano, Worcestershire, salt, and pepper. Mix together using your hands just until combined. Form the mixture into meatballs a bit larger than golf balls.

2. Heat the olive oil in a large nonstick skillet over medium-high heat. Add the meatballs and cook, turning, until browned, about 10 minutes. Transfer the meatballs to a plate.

3. Discard any oil from the pan. Add the tomato sauce, tomatoes, basil, and oregano to the pan, stir, and bring to a simmer. Gently place the meatballs in the sauce, cover, and simmer for 30 minutes, or until the meatballs are cooked through. Turn the meatballs about halfway through the cooking time.

4. Place slices of mozzarella on the meatballs and simmer for an additional 5 minutes, or until melted.

Note: Avoid leaner beef—the meatballs won't stick together as well. For the best taste, use 80 to 85 percent lean beef. Just make sure to drain off all excess fat during cooking or you'll have a "watery" sauce.

Fat-Burning Time Zone and Reloading Time Zone

SAUTÉED BABY ARTICHOKES

2   tablespoons lemon juice, plus more for sprinkling
1   package baby artichokes
1   cup chicken broth
2   tablespoons olive oil
1   teaspoon minced garlic
1   teaspoon dried basil
     Salt and freshly ground pepper to taste

1. Add the 2 tablespoons lemon juice to a bowl of water. For each artichoke, cut the stem off at the base. Peel off and discard the green petals until you reach the tender yellow ones. Cut off the top one-third of the artichoke. As you prepare the artichokes, drop them into the bowl of lemon water to prevent browning.

2. In a large skillet, bring the broth to boiling over medium-high heat. Add the artichokes, cover, and simmer for 3 to 5 minutes.

3. Transfer the artichokes to a bowl and discard the broth. In the same skillet, heat the olive oil over medium heat. Add the artichokes and garlic. Cook, stirring, until lightly browned, about 5 minutes. Sprinkle with the basil, lemon juice, and salt and pepper.

USDA researchers found that artichokes have more disease-fighting antioxidants than any other vegetable they tested. And the egg-size baby version allows you to eat the entire artichoke—heart and leaves—as you would a piece of broccoli. Look for them in the produce section of higher-end grocery stores; they're usually in a shrink-wrapped package.

Fat-Burning Time Zone

POT ROAST

       2   tablespoons olive oil
       1   chuck roast (2 to 2½ pounds)
           Salt and freshly ground pepper
    3–4   celery stalks, diced
       1   teaspoon chopped garlic
       1   can (8 ounces) tomato sauce
       1   tablespoon dried thyme
       1   tablespoon dried parsley
       2   cups beef broth
       2   cups red wine
       2   bay leaves
     1½   teaspoons Expert Foods ThickenThin not/Starch thickener (see note)

1. In a large pot, heat the olive oil over medium-high heat. Season both sides of the beef with salt and pepper. Place the beef in the pot and sear until browned, about 5 minutes each side. Remove from the pot and set aside.

2. In the same pot, combine the celery and garlic. Sauté for about 2 minutes, being careful not to burn the garlic. Add the tomato sauce, thyme, parsley, and 1 cup of the broth. Stir to combine.

3. Return the beef to the pot. Add the remaining broth, the wine, and the bay leaves. Bring to a boil. Cover, reduce the heat, and simmer for 2 to 3 hours. The longer you simmer, the more tender the beef will be.

4. Remove the meat from the pot. Cover and let rest for 10 to 15 minutes. Meanwhile, bring the liquid in the pot to a boil and add the thickener. Simmer for about 10 minutes, until the sauce thickens. Discard the bay leaves. Spoon the sauce over the meat and serve.

Note: ThickenThin not/Starch thickener (www.expertfoods.com) is an excellent low-carb replacement for flour when a recipe calls for a thicker sauce.

Fat-Burning Time Zone and Reloading Time Zone

ROASTED TURNIPS

2   medium-size turnips, cut into bite-size chunks
1   package (8 to 10 ounces) white button mushrooms, halved
2   cups pearl onions
    Salt and freshly ground pepper
2   tablespoons olive oil

1. Preheat the oven to 400°F.

2. Place the turnips, mushrooms, and onions in a large roasting pan. Season with salt and pepper and drizzle with the olive oil. (For extra flavor, stir in 2 tablespoons of liquid from the Pot Roast, page 125).

3. Roast the vegetables for 30 minutes, until they begin to brown on the edges.

Fat-Burning Time Zone

TUSCAN RIB-EYE STEAK AND PROSCIUTTO-WRAPPED ASPARAGUS

Marinade and Steak

- ¼ cup balsamic vinegar
  Juice of ½ lemon
- ¼ cup olive oil
- 1 tablespoon Dijon mustard
- 2 tablespoons rosemary
- 1 teaspoon chopped garlic
- 2 rib-eye steaks

Prosciutto-Wrapped Asparagus

- 1 bunch asparagus, ends trimmed
  Olive oil
  Freshly ground pepper
- 1 package (about 4 ounces) thin-sliced prosciutto

1. For the marinade and steak: Heat the grill or grill pan to medium-high heat.

2. In a small bowl, combine the vinegar, lemon juice, olive, oil, mustard, rosemary, and garlic and pour over the beef (in a plastic bag or low dish). Let marinate for at least 15 minutes.

3. Grill the steaks until desired doneness, about 6 to 7 minutes per side for medium-rare.

4. For the asparagus: Preheat oven to 385°F. Place the asparagus on a large baking sheet. Drizzle with the olive oil and season with the pepper. Mix with your hands until the asparagus is evenly covered.

5. Wrap 1 slice of prosciutto around 2 or 3 asparagus stalks. Return the bundle to the baking sheet. Repeat, evenly spacing the asparagus on the pan.

6. Bake for about 15 minutes, until the prosciutto starts crisping and the asparagus is al dente.

Reloading Time Zone

BURRITOS

1   pound ground beef
1   red bell pepper, sliced
1   package taco seasoning, plus water as directed on the package
     Whole grain tortillas
2   cups shredded Monterey Jack or Cheddar cheese
2   cups shredded romaine lettuce
2   cups diced tomatoes
     Salsa
1   teaspoon olive oil

1. Cook the beef in a large sauté pan over medium-high heat until browned. Add the red pepper and continue to cook, stirring, until softened slightly. Add the taco seasoning and water, stir, and simmer for 10 minutes, until the pepper slices are al dente.

2. Place a tortilla on a flat surface. Spoon 2 scoops of the beef mixture on the bottom one-third of the tortilla. Layer on cheese, lettuce, tomatoes, and salsa, being careful not to overload the tortilla. Fold the left and the right sides of the tortilla inward 1 inch, and then, starting from the bottom, roll up the tortilla until the seam is down. Repeat to make additional burritos.

3. Using a napkin or a paper towel, rub the olive oil on the bottom of a sauté pan. Heat on medium-high until hot but not smoking. Place the burritos, in batches if necessary, in the pan and cook for 3 to 4 minutes. Flip and cook on the other side for 3 to 4 minutes longer, until heated through and browned.

PART IV: TRAINING

CHAPTER 10

THE SCIENCE OF LIFTING

I f you pick up a heavy weight, put it down, and repeat a few times, and you do it often enough, you *will* build muscle. You will also burn calories. And you will raise your metabolism. All of which will help you lose fat, and better still, maintain that fat loss for the rest of your life. Sound simple? It is.

Yet you'll find that because there are so many ways to accomplish this simple task of picking up a heavy weight, putting it down, and repeating, there are hundreds if not thousands of opinions on how best to do it. And we imagine that they all "work." At least as long as you consistently use whatever protocol it is that's recommended.

But we aren't just interested in what works. We're interested in what works *best*. Or more specifically, what works best *and* fits into your lifestyle. That's because a training program is only effective if you actually have time to follow through with it. For instance, consider that British researchers recently determined that men who lifted weights 3 days a week for 5 weeks increased muscle size by about 0.2 percent per day. Sure, this amount of growth is unnoticeable from day to day. But imagine how dramatic the cumulative effect would be if you were to work all your major muscle groups 3 days a week, 52 weeks a year. This is called consistency, and it's the true key to achieving the most success possible on any exercise program.

So with fostering consistency in mind, we set out to create an overarching fitness philosophy that centers on achieving the best results in the least amount of time. The idea is simply that most of us don't have an hour or two to work out, 6 days a week. And even if we did, would that actually be optimal? After all, when it comes to building muscle, the law of diminishing returns always applies at some point. Case in point: Research shows that performing 1 set of an exercise works for building muscle, but that 2 sets work better. But what about, say, 10 sets? Is this better than doing 8 sets or even 4? These are the questions we asked when we created our fitness philosophy, and when we designed the TNT Workout Plan. For answers, we relied on more than 50 years of muscle research, and on the practical research of our friend and colleague, Alwyn Cosgrove, MS, CSCS. Cosgrove's a former world-class martial artist turned strength coach, who's now recognized as one of the country's foremost fitness experts.

Now Cosgrove doesn't claim to be a muscle scientist. But in a sense, he's become one by default. Since he opened his gym, Results Fitness, in 2000, he's kept a detailed account of every single session conducted. This effort was at first economically motivated: "Clients pay for the fastest results," he says. "So to compete with the gym down the street, I had to find out what works the best." And that meant collecting workout data on a large number of average men who were using a variety of different training methods.

Unlike commercial health clubs, Cosgrove's facility—located in Santa Clarita, California—offers only semiprivate training, meaning each workout is designed, monitored, and recorded by a member of the staff. Consider that in a typical week it hosts 400 workouts, providing feedback on 20,800 sessions a year. To equal those numbers, a regular guy would have to work out every single day for 57 years. In effect, that makes Cosgrove's gym a bona fide research laboratory. And his gym-rat clients, it seems, human lab rats. All of which underscores the real-world relevance of his findings.

To explain his observations, he's tried to bridge the academic research, like the kind we conduct in our laboratory at the University of Connecticut, with the practical application of exercises, sets, and repetitions. "A 19th-century English biologist named Thomas Huxley once said that 'science is nothing but organized common sense,'" explains Cosgrove. "Which is what training should be." We couldn't agree more.

In the pages that follow, we'll introduce you to the findings of Cosgrove's human experiment, as well as to how they mesh with the current scientific research. The end result is a weight-training philosophy that's not just gym-proven, it's supported by science.

And more importantly, it's highly practical, which will surely lead to greater consistency.

THE LOGIC OF TOTAL-BODY TRAINING

The biology of muscle isn't rocket science. At its most basic level is the SAID principle, an acronym for the *specific adaptation to imposed demand*. Think of this as the use-it-or-lose-it law. When a muscle fiber is exposed to a regular challenge, it makes structural adaptations in order to reduce stress on the body. In other words, it might grow bigger and stronger, or become more resistant to fatigue. Which is why you can perform everyday functions—like walking up the stairs or picking up a light object—with little effort.

Now let's apply the SAID principle to your workout. When you lift weights, you cause tiny tears in your muscle fibers, known as *microtrauma*. This muscle disruption accelerates a process we've already discussed—muscle protein synthesis. In this process, amino acids are used to repair and reinforce the fibers, making the fibers resistant to damage in the future. And although this happens at a microscopic level, the effect becomes visibly evident over time (assuming you have adequate nutrition)—in the form of bigger arms, broader shoulders, and a thicker chest. Consider it human adaptation at its finest. There's another benefit to this microtrauma: Repairing your muscles is an expensive metabolic process. That is, it requires calories, which results in raising your metabolism for hours after your workout is over. This is frequently referred to as the *afterburn effect*. It's important to note that the afterburn effect is unique to exercise that heavily challenges your muscles. So it doesn't occur with aerobic training, like when you run 4 or 5 miles at a steady pace.

Understanding all of this provides you with a logical rationale for how often you should train your muscles. In multiple studies over the last decade, researchers at the University of Texas Medical Branch in Galveston have reported that muscle protein synthesis is elevated for up to 48 hours after a resistance training session. So if you work out on Monday at 7 p.m., your body is in muscle-growth mode until Wednesday at 7 p.m. After 48 hours, though, the biological stimulus for your body to build new muscle returns to normal. Turns out, that's similar to the duration your metabolism is elevated after a heavy-lifting workout, too. For instance, University of Wisconsin scientists found that performing 12 total sets—4 sets each of the bench press, power clean, and squat—increased metabolism for 39 hours after the training session.

On paper, both of these findings support Cosgrove's first assertion: "Performing total-body workouts, three times a week, is the most effective way to gain muscle and lose fat." Unfortunately, that advice is in direct contradiction to what most guys actually do. That's because almost everyone subscribes to a leftover from the *Stay Hungry* days of weight lifting: what we call *body-part training*.

The idea is to divide the body into specific muscle groups, or body parts, and then to dedicate an entire training session to working just one part. For example, you might perform exercises for your chest on Monday, your back on Tuesday, your shoulders on Wednesday, and so on. The result is a workout regimen that typically requires 5 to 6 days a week. But even though you're training daily, each muscle group is only targeted once a week. So in essence, those muscles grow for just 2 days out of every 7. With total-body workouts, though, you can work each muscle more often. "By training a muscle three times a week, it spends more total time growing," says Cosgrove.

Science agrees. Anatomically speaking, you can't isolate muscle groups in the first place. Which is Cosgrove's other beef with body-part training. Imagine, for a moment, if you could strip the skin away from your muscles, exposing them to view. You'd clearly see that they're interconnected, surrounding the body like a unified web. This is because all of your muscles are enclosed in a tough connective tissue called *fascia*. And since fascia attaches to bone and other muscles, it creates "functional" relationships between seemingly separate muscle groups.

Even a small movement of your upper arm triggers a complicated network of muscles from your shoulder down to your hip. Here's why: Your latissimus dorsi (or *lats*), the largest muscle of your back, attaches to your upper arm bone, your shoulder blade, your spine, and your thoracolumbar fascia—a layer of deep tissue that connects to your spine and pelvis. Your glute, or rear hip muscle, attaches to your pelvis. See the connections?

This point isn't debatable; it's a scientific fact. "It's impossible to isolate a muscle with any exercise; you can't even pick up a pencil with just one muscle," says Cosgrove. Take the example of a popular exercise known as the bent-over row. If you subscribe to body-part training, it's a "back" exercise. But because of the interconnection between the muscles and connective tissues of the hips and back, your hamstrings and glutes are contracted for the entire exercise. So you're not only working your back, you're challenging your legs as well. And don't forget the involvement of your forearms and biceps in pulling the bar to your chest. "You can separate your workouts by muscle groups, but based on science, it's illogical," says Cosgrove. "You're not actually separating anything." Which is another reason that total-body training just makes good sense.

Of course, semantics aside, everyone acknowledges that you can *emphasize* a muscle group by choosing the appropriate exercises. However, since body-part training is generally performed intensely on consecutive days, it impedes the recovery process. The nutrients your body needs to repair muscle damage from the previous day are allocated toward providing energy for your workout instead. Fact is, your muscles grow best when your body is resting, not working. This isn't an issue with Cosgrove's total-body recommendation, since there's a built-in recovery day between each session.

THE TIME FACTOR

There is a practical argument against total-body training. If a typical chest workout takes 30 minutes or more to complete, you'd have to spend hours in the gym to work your entire body. "That's based on the assumption that a chest workout needs to take 30 minutes," says Cosgrove. He goes on to explain that a typical chest day might consist of 3 sets of four exercises, for a total of 12 sets. Keep in mind, that's the amount you would perform for the whole week. But Cosgrove says you could perform that same amount of work—12 total sets—in the same time period by doing 4 sets, 3 days a week. "I've found that training works like a prescription," says Cosgrove. "You wouldn't take an entire bottle of Advil on Monday to relieve pain all week; you'd take smaller doses at more regular intervals."

And a recent study at the University of Alabama supports this notion. The researchers had one group of men train each muscle group once a week for 3 months; another group performed the same number of total sets weekly, but split them up equally between three total-body workouts. The result? The men who lifted more frequently gained 9 pounds of muscle—5 more than those who only trained each muscle once a week.

But to save even more time, Cosgrove employs another strategy: alternating sets. When possible, he pairs exercises that work opposite muscle groups, and cuts the rest period between sets in half.

It's a concept based on the scientific work of Sir Charles Scott Sherrington, who won the Nobel Prize in 1932 for his contributions in the field of physiology and neuroscience. Sherrington's law of reciprocal inhibition states that "for every neural activation of a muscle, there is a corresponding inhibition of the opposing muscle." That means when you work your chest muscles, the corresponding back muscles are forced to relax, thereby resting.

So instead of waiting 2 minutes between sets of a bench press, you can perform 1 set of the bench press, rest for just 1 minute, and then do a bent-over row. After you finish, you'll rest again, and then repeat the entire process until you complete all sets of both exercises. "In an average workout, this technique saves at least 8 to 10 minutes," says Cosgrove. "And without sacrificing performance."

There's another piece to this puzzle, though. In analyzing thousands of workout logs, Cosgrove developed a volume-threshold theory. "It seems that growth occurs once a muscle has been exposed to 90 to 120 seconds of total tension," he says.

For an example, let's say it takes 5 seconds to complete 1 repetition. That means 1 set of 8 repetitions would place your muscles under tension for 40 seconds. So using Cosgrove's theory, you'd only need to do 3 sets—a total of 120 seconds—to perform enough exercise to stimulate muscle growth. Likewise with 4 sets of 5 repetitions, or 2 sets of 12 repetitions.

However, even Cosgrove insists this is more theory than fact. Call it an original hypothesis, and primarily for one reason: Human studies simply haven't compared a wide variety of set and repetition ranges, or even controlled for the duration of muscle tension. So there's simply no data to draw from. At least, not until you look elsewhere in the animal kingdom.

You see, some men simply gain muscle faster, easier, and to a greater degree than others, which is why scientists study rats. Rats, unlike humans, are a homogenous species, meaning there's little variation from one to another. And that allows scientists to study more accurately the enzymes, metabolic pathways, and genes that regulate muscle growth.

Of course, actual lab rats aren't gym rats by nature. So in 1992, a team of researchers at the University of California, Irvine, developed a rat-sized resistance training apparatus—a device that looks like a high-tech leg curl machine. However, since they couldn't simply ask a group of rats to lift weights, or even know how much effort one is exerting, there was another step involved.

The researchers permanently implanted a stainless steel wire in the gastrocnemius muscle of each rat's hind limb, and ran the wire under the skin to the skull, where two small screws had been inserted using a handheld drill. By connecting an electrode to the outside of the screws, the scientists were then able to manually stimulate the muscle with an electric current, causing it to contract with maximal force. This allowed them to mimic a human weight-lifting workout, complete with sets and repetitions.

To find out if it worked, the rats were "encouraged" to perform 4 sets of 10 repetitions, with each repetition lasting 2 seconds—a total tension time of 80 seconds. The results were disappointing: The group didn't increase muscle size in an 8-week period. Which either meant that the machine didn't work or that the volume of exercise was too low. So the researchers tweaked the workout. When the contractions were increased to 4 seconds in duration, doubling the total tension time, the rats gained a significant amount of muscle mass—and in just 4 weeks, not 8.

Of course, this doesn't authoritatively validate Cosgrove's volume-threshold theory in humans, but it does provide a biological precedence that supports it. And it just may be that some of his data is simply ahead of its time.

THE MORE MUSCLE SECRET

"Go heavy or go home" is a common saying among bodybuilders. And while it's crucial that you use a weight that provides a challenging load, the mantra is flawed. That's because muscle fibers can grow in two ways. The first is when myofibrils—the parts of the fiber that contain the contractile proteins—increase in number and density. This type of growth leads to strength gains and can by accomplished by using heavy weights that only allow 1 to 7 repetitions.

The second type of growth, however, occurs when your muscles are forced to contract for longer periods of time. Typically, that means using lighter loads that allow you to complete 12 to 15 repetitions. Think of it as improving the endurance of the muscle fiber. This increases the number of energy-producing structures within the muscle fiber, increasing its size. So you don't get significantly stronger, but you do get bigger. (One note: Although experienced lifters won't build much strength in the 12- to 15-repetition range, beginners will—and we'll explain why a little later in this chapter.)

Using a repetition range that falls between the two causes a combination of both types of growth, but each to a lesser degree. And that's why Cosgrove uses all 3 repetition ranges. For instance, he might prescribe 5 repetitions for each exercise on Monday, 10 repetitions on Wednesday, and 15 repetitions on Friday. "It not only leads to better growth, but it helps to keep from hitting plateaus," says Cosgrove.

And indeed, in a 2003 study, Arizona State University researchers discovered that men who alternated their repetition ranges in each of three weekly training sessions—a technique called *undulating periodization*—gained twice as much strength as men who performed the same number of repetitions every workout. To Cosgrove, it's just another of case of a logical approach generating a logical result.

TRANSLATING PHILOSOPHY TO PRACTICE

The take-home message from all of this, of course, is that the most effective workout isn't necessarily the longest or the hardest; it's simply the smartest. And think about it: By training smarter, you can exercise for less total time each week, which will likely result in greater consistency. "Building muscle and losing fat take sweat, guts, and determination," says Cosgrove. "So why make it harder than it needs to be?" We can't think of a single reason. Can you?

Assuming the answer is no, you should now have a solid understanding of the basic philosophy we've used to create the TNT Workout Plan. It's simple, effective, and ultimately, it just makes good sense. But a philosophy is just that. For example, you can see that a total-body workout, done 3 days a week, with varying repetition ranges, is an effective way to train, but perhaps you'd like to know about all the other details. Like, how do all the individual parts come together to create a cohesive workout plan? And what about cardio? Where does that fit in? These are all good questions, which is why we've provided the details on how we determined each parameter of the TNT Workout Plan. Consider it your guide to building the perfect workout—one that will provide you with the knowledge to perhaps create a training plan of your own down the line. Or more importantly, become a better judge of workouts that you find in magazines, on the Internet, and in other books.

HOW WE DESIGNED
THE TNT WORKOUT PLAN

CHOOSING THE REPETITIONS

Of all the workout variables—including exercise selection—the number of repetitions was actually the first one that we determined. The reason is that the number of repetitions dictates how your muscles are going to adapt. As we've already explained, heavy weights and low repetitions increase muscle size differently than lighter weights and higher repetitions.

But there's another factor, and that's experience level. People who haven't lifted weights before have a poorly developed neuromuscular system. Your neuromuscular system is composed of all your muscle fibers and all the nerves that activate those muscle fibers. And the command center of all of this is your central nervous system, which includes your brain and spinal cord. In simple terms, this is how your brain communicates with your muscles, what's commonly referred to as the mind-muscle connection.

Now, if you haven't practiced an exercise or movement before, you won't be very good at it. Picture someone trying to shoot a basketball for the first time. Typically, he'll look uncoordinated, especially compared to someone who's been playing for years. However, with enough practice, he'll start to improve. It's the same way with weight training. If you've never performed a dumbbell bench press before, it'll be very awkward, and you won't be able to handle much weight. This is because your mind isn't used to telling your muscles—via your nerves—how to perform this movement. As a result, it's not able to activate a high number of muscle fibers, which prevents you from using heavier dumbbells.

However, after a few workouts, your mind-muscle connection will improve dramatically, and because of this, so will your strength and your ability to control the weight. This is why beginners often double their strength in just a few weeks after starting a lifting program. It's also why they're better off sticking with higher repetitions when they initiate a lifting routine. The idea is that, to improve the mind-muscle connection as fast as possible, they need practice—so more repetitions are better than fewer repetitions. In fact, Arizona State University researchers found that beginners achieved the best gains in strength when they performed 12 to 15 repetitions. And as they improved, they needed heavier weights and lower repetitions to continue gaining strength.

This knowledge provided us with a starting place for phase 1 of the Get Back in Shape Workout. If you look closely at the workouts as a whole, you'll see that the first 4-week workout is performed by doing 15 repetitions (with one exception) for each set. Then, as we progress from phase to phase, the repetitions are manipulated to create different adaptations. This is called *periodization,* and it's a scientifically proven way to organize and vary a workout plan to ensure maximal gains, and avoid plateaus. Ultimately, when you reach the Advanced Workout, you'll be ready for the aforementioned *undulating periodization*—where you alternate your repetitions with each training session—to achieve the best results possible.

DETERMINING THE NUMBER OF SETS

The number of sets we chose, for the most part, was based on the number of repetitions performed in each workout. This allowed us to put into practice the concept of total time under tension. In the workout section, you'll find that we've recommended that each repetition take 5 seconds to perform—3 seconds to lower, a 1-second pause in the middle, and 1 second to lift. So to calculate total time under tension, we just had to multiply the number of repetitions prescribed by 5 seconds. Then we added on enough sets to hit 90 to 120 seconds of total tension time.

Another way to look at this is that total repetitions of each exercise should stay in the 25- to 50-repetition range. (Example: If you do 3 sets of 10 reps, you've performed 30 total repetitions.) We don't have science to prove this, but as a general rule, it seems to work very well.

In either case—using total tension time or total repetitions—the number of sets comes out nearly the same. So as a basic guideline, if you're doing higher repetitions, you'll do fewer sets; if you're doing lower repetitions, you'll do more sets. This ensures that you're forcing your muscles to work equally hard—although in different ways—in each workout.

The one caveat to all of this, particularly in the Get Back in Shape Workout, is that we wanted to ensure that there was an adequate amount of exercise to challenge conditioning levels. So in the first phase, we start out with just 2 sets for each exercise, but progress to 4 sets by the end of phase 2. In some cases, this leads to an even higher amount of total tension time than is *needed* for muscle growth. However, this extra work isn't performed in vain. It's intended to increase the total work performed, in order to ramp up the fat loss and overall conditioning effects of the workout.

DECIDING ON REST PERIODS

The amount of time you rest between sets is a crucial, but often overlooked, factor in most workouts. It works like this: The longer you rest, the more fully your muscle fibers can recover between sets. This allows you to work more total muscle fibers each set, leading to growth. However, shorter rest periods train your muscles to recover faster, which helps increase their size, too. To create a balance, we use a simple system: The lower your repetitions—and heavier the weights—the longer you rest between sets; the higher your repetitions—and lighter the weights—the shorter your rest. Why? When you lift heavy weights, you're recruiting fast-twitch muscle fibers, which are the fibers that generate the most force, but also fatigue the fastest and take the longest to recover. So giving them ample time to rest helps ensure you train them fully each set. When you use lighter weights and do more repetitions, you're mainly hitting your slow-twitch muscle fibers. These are not only more resistant to fatigue than fast-twitch fibers, but they recover much more quickly, too. Which means that, even after a challenging high-rep set, they're ready for a repeat performance in a short period of time.

By pairing this systematic approach with the time-saving alternating-sets method, we've minimized the amount of rest needed between every set, while maximizing the amount of weight that you can lift in each exercise. This is a key factor in stimulating the most muscle growth in the least amount of time possible. For this reason, we recommend that you use a digital watch during your workouts, in order to closely adhere to the prescribed rest periods.

SELECTING THE EXERCISES

To start, we focused on compound exercises. Compound exercises are those that require you to move at more than one joint—the bench press, squat, row, and lunge are a few examples. These work far more muscles than isolation exercises such as the arm curl or triceps extension, which require that you move at only one joint. In fact, you'll notice that we didn't include one arm curl or triceps extension—both of which are the staples of most guys' workouts—in the TNT Workout Plan. The reason is simple: When you have a limited amount of time to work out, you need to use the exercises that will provide the *most* benefits to your body. To include a few sets of arm curls in a 30-minute workout would have been at the expense of a compound exercise, and that doesn't make sense, particularly from an efficiency standpoint. For example, the row is a compound exercise that works the muscles of your back *and* biceps; the arm curl only trains your biceps.

Of course, you may say, "Who cares! I want to do arm curls." To which we reply: Great. Just do them *after* you've completed all of the other exercises in your workout. Trust us, arm curls won't help you lose fat, and they won't help you build nearly as much muscle as rows. What's more, your arms will grow plenty without them, using the exercises that we've prescribed throughout our plan. However, if you're convinced you need arm curls and triceps extensions and have the extra time, go ahead and tack them on to the end of your training session.

Now besides focusing on compound movements, the other main factor we considered when choosing exercises was balance. For simplicity, you might first think of this in body-part terms. The concept being that we want to do an equal amount of work for both the chest and the back. Trouble is, this is another flaw with body-part training. That's because the muscles of your back are many, and they have many different functions, compared to your chest, which mainly consists of one large muscle group, commonly called the *pecs*. (This is an oversimplification, of course, but it works as an example.) Training your chest and your back with an equal number of sets would either result in overworking your chest or underworking your back—or both.

The solution to this problem is to stop categorizing exercises according to muscle groups and body parts. Instead, we use *movement patterns,* a technique first popularized by Australian strength coach Ian King just a few years ago. By thinking in terms of movement patterns—and not body parts—we can more effectively balance our training, and our bodies. The result is better performance in all exercises, a more symmetrical physique, and a lower risk of injuries in the future.

So what is this exactly? It's the classification of exercises into six movement patterns: Horizontal Press, Horizontal Pull, Vertical Press, Vertical Pull, Quadriceps-Dominant, and Hip-Dominant. Here's a summary of each:

Horizontal Press: Upper body exercises in which you move the weight away from your torso horizontally. The trick to identifying these exercises is to imagine that your torso is upright when doing them. Examples: pushups, dips, or any type of bench press.

Horizontal Pull: Upper body exercises that require you to move the weight toward your torso horizontally. Again, picture your torso in an upright position to determine the movement pattern. Examples: any type of row, such as the bent-over row or seated row.

Vertical Press: Upper body exercises that require you to move the weight in an upward direction in relation to your upright torso. Examples: scaption and any type of shoulder press.

Vertical Pull: Exercises that require you to move the weight (or bar) in a downward direction in relation to your upright torso. Examples: lat pulldowns, pullovers, and any type of pullup or chinup.

Quadriceps-Dominant: Lower body exercises in which your quadriceps are the primary mover. Rule of thumb: If your torso is vertical or bent forward less than 45 degrees, consider the exercise Quad-Dominant. (This is only true when your upper body is actively involved in the exercise—for instance, holding the bar or dumbbell during lunges.) Examples: any type of squat or lunge.

Hip-Dominant: Exercises in which your hamstrings or glutes are the primary movers. An easy way to judge: If your torso is bent forward more than 45 degrees, classify it as Hip-Dominant (unless your upper body has no involvement, such as on the Swiss-ball leg curl). Examples: stepups, Swiss-ball leg curl, hip extension, back extension, and any type of deadlift.

Knowing this, the most basic way to create a balanced workout is to do an equal number of sets for each upper body movement pattern and an equal number of sets for each lower body movement pattern. For instance, if you do 3 sets of the bench press (Horizontal Press), you'll also want to do 3 sets of the bent-over row (Horizontal Pull), 3 sets of pullups (Vertical Pull), and 3 sets of the shoulder press (Vertical Press).

However, to truly balance your workout, you have to look at other factors, such as the amount of loading that occurs in each movement pattern. For example, within a workout, you ideally want to lift an equal amount of total weight—known as the *volume* of work that's performed—for each upper body movement pattern and, separately, each lower body movement pattern. (To calculate volume, multiply the number of sets by repetitions and then multiply that number by the amount of weight used.) So if your volume for a specific Horizontal Press exercise is significantly more than that of your Horizontal Pull, or even Vertical Pull, your workout isn't balanced. To rectify this, you might do a fewer number of sets or repetitions of the Horizontal Press, or add another Horizontal Pull exercise. If you look closely, you'll see examples of this throughout the TNT Workout Plan. Creating this type of balance isn't always possible in a specific 4-week workout, but throughout an entire 12-week plan, for instance, it should be in the ballpark across all the movement patterns.

Of course, we don't tell you this because it's necessary for you to understand it to achieve all the benefits from our program. But we hope that it's useful for you to realize how much thought has gone into creating the TNT Workout Plan. There's also an immediate benefit: Because you now understand movement patterns, you can substitute exercises throughout the program if necessary. For example, if a workout calls for a seated row—a Horizontal Pull movement—but you don't have access to a seated row machine, you can simply swap in another Horizontal Pull that matches your equipment. Obviously, we'd advise you to stick with the plan as shown, but when that's not practical, this is a smart way to adjust the program.

Also, we should point out that there are a few other movement patterns. For instance, you can separate core exercises into six movement patterns, too: trunk flexion, trunk extension, trunk rotation, hip flexion, hip extension, and hip rotation. However, to keep everything as simple as possible, we'll just refer to these movements as core exercises. And just to satisfy any lingering curiosity, biceps curls fall into the category of *elbow flexion* while triceps extensions are classified as *elbow extension*.

THE QUESTION OF CARDIO

Because you may be wondering, we felt it necessary to address why we don't emphasize "cardio," or more appropriately, aerobic exercise. The main reason is that aerobic exercise isn't very effective for fat loss. In fact, it's not needed at all, especially when you're closely following the TNT Diet. For example, in a 2007 study, Louisiana State University researchers reported that over-weight men who simply dieted lost the same amount of fat as those who both dieted and performed aerobic exercise 45 minutes a day, 5 days a week. This was similar to what we found in our laboratory, when dieters lost the same amount of fat as those who dieted and performed aerobic exercise, a study we describe in detail in Chapter 1.

That said, you may want to perform aerobic exercise for its health benefits. And if that's the case, we only encourage you. However, we'd like to point out that the weight-training workouts you'll be performing will provide you with many of the same health benefits, cardiovascular and others, as aerobic activity—particularly for the time involved. As such, there's no reason for

---

The Anatomy of Muscle

Sarcomere: Thousands of tiny proteins that contract under electrical stimulation within a muscle cell

Myofibril: A chain of sarcomeres that together generate force to help a cell contract

Sarcoplasm: A semifluid membrane that surrounds the muscle fiber and contains structures—such as mitochondria—that provide energy for muscular contraction

Muscle fiber: A single muscle cell, which contains several hundred to several thousand myofibrils

Fascicle: A bundle of several muscle fibers

Muscle: A bundle of fascicles that are enclosed in a sheath of connective tissue called *fascia*

Tendon: Tough connective tissue that attaches the muscle to the bone

Capillaries: Tiny blood vessels that deliver nutrients and enzymes to the muscle fiber

you to feel like you're missing out. If you have the time, though, and want an efficient cardio workout, we've provided this as an option. You'll notice that the workouts contain no steady-state aerobic exercise, only high-intensity intervals. Why? Because research shows that intervals are the most efficient way to improve your aerobic fitness, and they're also far more effective for reducing your glycogen levels. So keeping with our overall fitness philosophy, it only makes sense for us to recommend this approach.

TNT TRANSFORMATION

"My pants and shirts are too big."

Name: **Paul Zaras**
Age: **37**
Height: **5 feet 10 inches**
Weight before: **219**
Weight after: **201**

PAUL ZARAS, AN E-COMMERCE ANALYST, became motivated to make a lifestyle change after seeing himself in a three-way mirror: "I looked like a big tub of goo." But like most people, he needed something simple, or as he so specifically put it: "A quick and dirty method that a nearing-middle-age guy could use to change the course of his physique."

So we sent him TNT, and Paul immediately began losing weight, dropping 7 pounds in the first 2 weeks. Then it got interesting: Thanksgiving arrived—along with a slew of holiday celebrations. "The timing of the year was the most challenging, but as long as I kept to my workouts, I was able to enjoy the holidays."

Even though Paul occasionally deviated from the plan—"You gotta live, right?"—he kept losing weight by sticking with his workouts and adhering to the diet guidelines *most* of the time. "I followed the 80 percent rule until after New Year's," he says. "Then I went back to the plan full bore."

Besides downsizing his wardrobe due to an 18-pound (and still falling) weight loss, Paul has also discovered an interesting side effect: "I feel like I can handle stress better, and my work productivity has increased." We say: Enjoy your raise, pal.

CHAPTER 11

THE TNT WORKOUT PLAN

If there's a common flaw in most workout plans, it's that, typically, there's no actual *plan* involved. Instead, there's just a collection of individual workouts, which upon close inspection, often look as if they could have been randomly thrown together. And in many cases, they probably were. The idea being that simply changing up your routine a little every 3 or 4 weeks will "shock" your muscles into growing, or help you break through a fat-loss plateau. But while that approach is certainly better than doing the same workout for months on end, it's hardly optimal—and it doesn't qualify as a *plan*. At least not an effective one.

No, for a plan to be truly effective, each workout must smartly build on the one before. This is called *progression,* and it's the key strategy for achieving the best results in the least amount of time. And, of course, it's the very strategy we used to design the TNT Workout Plan. See, progression requires that every detail—every exercise, set, repetition, and rest period—be carefully determined ahead of time, in the same manner you would if you were writing how-to instructions for building a new house.

So with that in mind, consider the TNT Workout Plan your how-to instructions for building a new *body.* Although it may look simplistic, you can be sure that each component of each workout has been rigorously scrutinized, and as a result, plays a crucial role in helping you lose fat and build muscle as fast as possible.

THINGS TO KNOW BEFORE YOU START . . .

There are two main components of the TNT Workout Plan: the dynamic warmup and the weight workouts. However, we've also included a cardio workout as an optional component. Here's an overview of each.

THE DYNAMIC WARMUP

To prepare your body for each workout session, you'll start with a 5-minute "dynamic" warmup. Essentially, a dynamic warmup is a series of body-weight exercises and calisthenics. Its first purpose is to increase blood flow to—or "warm"—every muscle in your body. This makes it far superior to simply warming up on the treadmill or stationary bike, which only increases blood flow to the muscles of your lower body.

In addition, a dynamic warmup stimulates your central nervous system. This is important because your central nervous system—your brain and spinal cord—is the control center for your muscles. By engaging it prior to a challenging weight workout, you'll improve the communication between your mind and muscles. The result of which is that you'll recruit more muscle fibers, allowing you to lift more weight.

It's also a great technique to use before you do other activities, such as sports. For instance, scientists at the United States Military Academy found that performing a dynamic workout before tests of athletic prowess helped men sprint faster, jump higher, and throw harder.

The other benefit of a dynamic warmup is that it's one of the best ways to improve your flexibility. Besides making you more mobile in everyday life, this allows you to perform exercises through a greater range of motion, which means you'll work more muscle during each repetition.

Now, to make our dynamic warmup even more useful, we asked Bill Hartman, PT, CSCS, one of the world's top physical therapists and strength coaches, to create a routine that not only optimally prepares your body for each workout but also addresses many of the muscle imbalances and weaknesses that plague the average guy. For instance, many men who sit at a desk all day share common problems, such as a slumped posture and a poor ability to activate the muscles of their hips and glutes. Early on, these factors might go unnoticed or simply cause a little nagging pain—such as an achy neck, back, or hips. Or they might lead to an injury, like a torn rotator cuff or hamstring pull.

But left unaddressed for the long term, these problems eventually result in debilitating muscle dysfunctions that make it difficult to do almost everything—including walk. Ever see a bent-over elderly man who can barely shuffle along, or worse yet, requires a walker? This is often caused not only by weak muscles but also from years of sitting and slumping. Which is why the dynamic warmup that Hartman created does more than just help you achieve a better workout; it can actually help keep you healthy for years down the road.

Of course, you'll probably be tempted to skip the dynamic warmup and move straight to the workout, despite all the benefits the warmup offers. But what's the upside of forgoing it—that you'll save 5 minutes? Think of it this way: We didn't include this dynamic warmup for any reason other than it will improve your workout, your body, and your results. And isn't that your goal?

To complete the dynamic warmup, you'll simply perform each exercise in the order shown (page 153) in a circuit, moving from one movement to the next without resting. Once you've completed all 10 exercises, you're ready to begin your weight workout.

THE WEIGHT WORKOUTS

The weight workouts have been divided into two 12-week programs, each of which comprises three 4-week phases. The first 12-week program is designed specifically for guys who have never lifted before, haven't lifted weights in more than 3 months, or have more than 10 pounds of fat to lose. We call this the Get Back in Shape Workout because that's exactly what it is. It's designed not only to burn fat, raise your metabolism, and stimulate muscle growth, but also to improve your overall physical conditioning. Which means that even if you're a longtime lifter who's laid off the weights for a couple of months, this is the program you should follow. In fact, we encourage everyone to start here.

The second 12-week program is the Advanced Workout. It requires the use of heavier weights, demands a higher base level of conditioning, and is more focused on building muscle and strength than the Get Back in Shape Workout. That doesn't mean it won't help you burn fat and elevate your metabolism. The emphasis of this program is geared to the guy who's already in shape—at least conditioning-wise—and wants to maximize muscle size. The key, though, is that the Advanced Workout was created as the next progression from the Get Back in Shape Workout. So once you complete the 12-week Get Back in Shape Workout, you can transition seamlessly into the Advanced Workout. In effect, this provides you with a 24-week workout plan.

To perform all of the workouts found in this chapter, follow these guidelines:

• Complete three weight-training workouts each week, resting at least a day between each session. So you might lift weights on Monday, Wednesday, and Friday, or on Tuesday, Thursday, and Saturday.

• Alternate between workouts, regardless of which phase of the program you're in. For instance, if the phase you're in consists of Workout A and Workout B, and you plan to lift on Monday, Wednesday, and Friday, you'd do Workout A on Monday, Workout B on Wednesday, and Workout A again on Friday. The next week, you'd do Workout B on Monday and Friday, and Workout A on Wednesday.

If the phase has three separate workouts—for example, Workout A, Workout B, and Workout C—you'll simply do Workout A on Monday, Workout B on Wednesday, and Workout C on Friday. Again, the idea is to rotate the workouts, so that you never complete the same workout in successive training sessions.

• Always do the exercises in the order shown in the chart. You'll perform the exercises using one of two techniques: straight sets or alternating sets.

  • Straight sets will be designated simply as a number—for instance, 1 or 3. Each time you see this, do 1 set of the exercise, rest for the prescribed amount of time, and then do another set. Complete all sets of the exercise before moving on to the next.

  • Alternating sets will be designated as a number and letter pair—for instance, 1A and 1B, and 2A and 2B. For these, perform 1 set of the first exercise, rest for the prescribed amount of time, then do 1 set of the second exercise and rest again. Then repeat the entire process. So if you're doing exercises 1A and 1B with a 60-second rest, you'll do 1 set of 1A, rest 60 seconds, then 1 set of 1B, and rest another 60 seconds. Continue alternating back and forth until you've completed all sets of both exercises.

• Unless otherwise noted in the exercise descriptions (which appear in alphabetical order in this chapter), complete all of the exercises in this manner:

  • Take about 3 seconds to lower the weight in a slow, controlled fashion. Ideally, you'll lower the weight at about the same rate of speed from top to bottom.

  • Pause momentarily in the "down" position or the midpoint of the lift. This is indicated in each exercise description.

  • Lift the weight as fast as you can while maintaining control of the bar or dumbbells.

  • On some exercises, like the lat pulldown, it will seem like the lowering portion is actually the part of the lift in which your muscles are contracting. But keep in mind that as you pull the bar down, the weight stack is actually rising. Don't worry; we'll indicate the speed at which you should perform each portion of the lift in every exercise description.

• For each exercise, choose the *heaviest* weight that allows you to complete all of the prescribed repetitions. Remember, the number of repetitions, and the speed at which you perform them, dictate the type of adaptations your muscles make. But you might also think of it this way: Prescribing a specific number of repetitions is just a way of instructing you how much weight to use. The lower the repetitions, the heavier the weight. And vice versa. For instance, if you can lift a weight 15 times, it's not going to do your muscles much good to lift it only 5 times. And if you choose a weight that's difficult to lift 5 times, there's no way you can pump out 15 repetitions.

So how do you figure out the right amount? Trial and error for the most part. You just have to make an educated guess and experiment. This is second nature for experienced lifters, but if you're new to training, don't stress over it; you'll catch on fast. The key is to get in there and start lifting. If you choose a weight that's too heavy or too light, just adjust it accordingly in your next set.

One simple way to gauge how close you are to the right weight is noting when you start to struggle with the weight. For example, if you're doing 10 repetitions, and all 10 seem easy, then the weight you're using is too light. If, however, you start to struggle on your 10th repetition, you've chosen the correct poundage. What does "start to struggle" mean? It's when the speed at which you can lift the weight slows. Some people call this the sticking point. Although you can push through it for another rep or two, the struggle indicates that your muscles have just about had it. This is also the point when most people start to "cheat" by changing their body posture to help them lift the weight. Again, the idea is to complete all of the repetitions in each set, while challenging your muscles maximally. Using the "start-to-struggle" concept is one way to help you do that.

OPTIONAL: THE CARDIO WORKOUT

Remember, this cardio workout isn't necessary to experience all of the benefits of the TNT Diet that you've read about so far. But it certainly provides health perks and will also improve your overall conditioning level. The plan is simple: It's a high-intensity interval workout that consists of short sprints of 30 to 60 seconds interspersed with longer periods of less-intensive activity. You can do the workout 2 to 3 days a week, outside or in the gym, preferably on the days between your weight workouts. If that isn't convenient, you can also tack the workouts on to the end of your weight-training session. Running is the optimal mode if you choose to exercise outside; a stationary bike will work best if you perform the workout in the gym.

Alternate between Workout A and Workout B each time you perform a cardio session. So if you lift on Monday, Wednesday, and Friday, you might do the Interval Workout A on Tuesday, and Interval Workout B on Thursday. Before each workout, warm up and cool down for 5 minutes at a slow, easy pace. To perform the intervals, run or cycle at the fastest pace you can maintain for the duration of the sprint time. Then slow down to a pace that's about 30 percent of your full effort for the recovery time. For instance, if you're running outside, this recovery pace might amount to a walk or a slow jog. Repeat until you've completed all of the prescribed intervals for each workout. Note that we've provided guidelines for the first 4 weeks. Once you've completed this 4-week plan, you can progress by sticking with the same number of total intervals (six in Workout A; five in Workout B), but decrease your recovery time by 5 to 10 seconds each week. If you stick with it long enough, you'll ultimately be sprinting and resting the same amount of time.

WORKOUT	SPRINT TIME	RECOVERY TIME	WEEK	INTERVALS
A	30 sec	90 sec	1 and 2	4
			3 and 4	6
B	60 sec	180 sec	1 and 2	3
			3 and 4	5

THE DYNAMIC WARMUP

HOW TO DO IT:

Without resting, perform 1 set of 10 repetitions of each exercise in the order shown. For each exercise, start slowly and gradually increase the speed that you perform the movement, while maintaining your form and complete control over your body at all times.

1. JUMPING JACKS

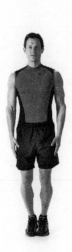 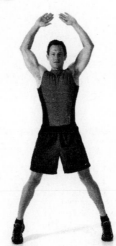

1. Stand with your feet together and your hands at your sides.

2. Simultaneously raise your arms above your head and jump up just enough to spread your feet.

3. Without pausing, quickly reverse the movement and repeat until you've completed 10 repetitions.

2. ARM CIRCLES

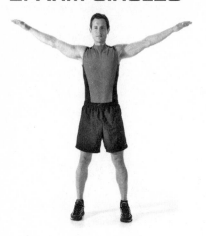 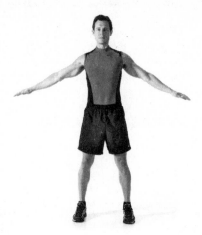

1. Stand, holding your arms straight out to your sides so that they're parallel to the floor.

2. Start by making small circles with your arm, progressing to bigger circles. Do 10 repetitions forward and 10 repetitions backward.

3. LUNGE

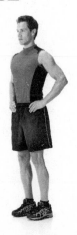 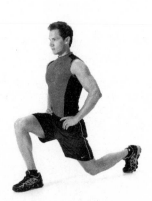

1. Stand with your feet shoulder width apart and your hands on your hips.

2. Step forward with your right leg and lower your body until your front knee is bent 90 degrees and your rear knee nearly touches the floor. Your front lower leg should be perpendicular to the floor and your torso should remain upright.

3. Push yourself back up to the starting position as quickly as you can and repeat with your left leg. That's 1 repetition. Do a total of 10 repetitions.

4. BODY-WEIGHT SQUAT

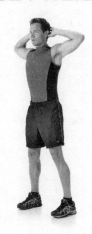
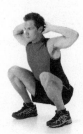

1. Stand with your feet spread slightly wider than your hips, and place your hands behind your head.

2. Lower your body as far as you can by pushing your hips back and bending your knees. Your back should be flat or slightly arched for the entire movement, and your lower legs should remain nearly perpendicular to the floor.

3. Pause, then return to the starting position. Do 10 repetitions.

5. HIP EXTENSION

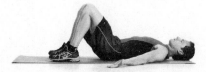
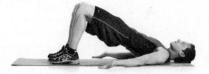

1. Lie on your back on the floor with your knees bent and your feet flat on the floor. Place your arms out to your sides at a 45-degree angle, your palms facing up.

2. Raise your hips so your body forms a straight line from your shoulders to your knees.

3. Lower your body back to the starting position. Do 10 repetitions.

6. LYING STRAIGHT-LEG RAISE

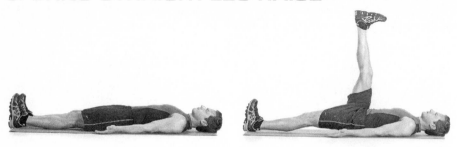

1. Lie on your back with your legs straight.

2. Keeping both knees straight, raise your right leg upward as far as possible. (Imagine that you're trying to kick a ball that's hanging over your body.) Complete 10 repetitions with your right leg, and then repeat with your left leg.

7. PUSHUP PLUS

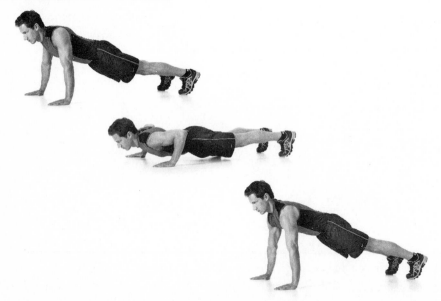

1. Get into pushup position—your hands slightly wider and in line with your shoulders—with your body forming a straight line from your ankles to your shoulders.

2. Quickly lower yourself until your upper arms are lower than your elbows, then push yourself back up.

3. Once your arms are straight again, push your torso upward without moving any other part of your body. (You'll rise up another couple of inches.) Pause momentarily, then perform another pushup. Do 10 repetitions.

8. THORACIC ROTATION

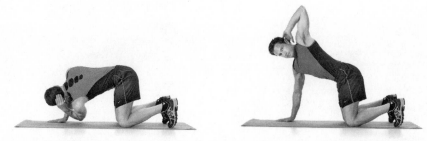

1. Get down on the floor on all fours. Then take your left hand and place it behind your head. Bend your upper back downward by pointing your left elbow at your right knee. This is the starting position.

2. While bracing your abs, raise your elbow toward the ceiling by rotating your upper back up and to the left as far as possible. (Bracing your abs—as if you're about to be punched in the gut—is important because it ensures that the rotation takes place at your upper back, and not your lower back.) Do 10 repetitions, then repeat on the other side, this time with your right hand placed on your head.

9. FIRE HYDRANT IN-OUT

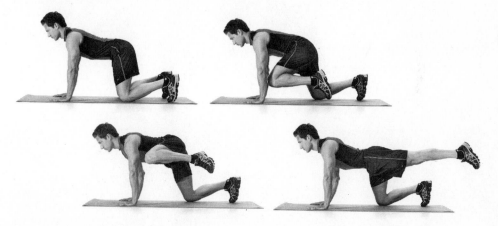

1. Get down on the floor on all fours.

2. To start the movement, pull your left knee as close as you can toward your chest.

3. Then raise it out to the side (like a dog at a fire hydrant).

4. Finally, kick your raised left leg straight back until it's in line with your torso.

5. Do 10 repetitions, and then repeat the movement with your right leg.

6. Next, perform 10 repetitions of the movement with each leg again, only this time, perform it in reverse order: Kick your leg straight back, bring it out the side, and then pull it toward your chest.

10. GROINERS

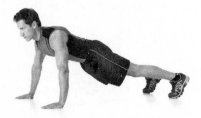 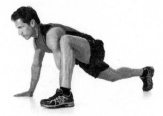

1. Get into pushup position—your hands slightly wider and in line with your shoulders—with your body forming a straight line from your ankles to your shoulders.

2. Now bring your left foot forward and place it next to and outside of your left hand for a brief moment.

3. Return to the starting position and repeat with your right leg. That's 1 repetition. Do a total of 10 repetitions.

THE GET BACK IN SHAPE WORKOUT

PHASE 1: WEEKS 1 THROUGH 4
WORKOUT A

ORDER	EXERCISE	REPS	SETS				REST (IN SEC)			
			Week 1	Week 2	Week 3	Week 4	Week 1	Week 2	Week 3	Week 4
1A	Static Lunge	15	2	2	3	3	45	45	45	30
1B	Incline Dumbbell Bench Press	12	2	2	3	3	45	45	45	30
2A	Hip Extension	15	2	2	3	3	45	45	45	30
2B	Seated Row to Neck	15	2	2	3	3	45	45	45	30
3	Prone Cobra	60 sec	1	1	1	1	—	—	—	—

WORKOUT B

ORDER	EXERCISE	REPS	SETS				REST (IN SEC)			
			Week 1	Week 2	Week 3	Week 4	Week 1	Week 2	Week 3	Week 4
1A	Dumbbell Stepup	15	2	2	3	3	45	45	45	30
1B	Neutral-Grip Shoulder Press	15	2	2	3	3	45	45	45	30
2A	Goblet Squat	15	2	2	3	3	45	45	45	30
2B	Dumbbell Pullover	15	2	2	3	3	45	45	45	30
3	Plank	60 sec	1	1	1	1	—	—	—	—

PHASE 2: WEEKS 5 THROUGH 8
WORKOUT A

ORDER	EXERCISE	REPS	SETS				REST (IN SEC)			
			Week 1	Week 2	Week 3	Week 4	Week 1	Week 2	Week 3	Week 4
1A	Wide-Grip Seated Row	12	3	3	4	4	45	30	45	30
1B	Romanian Deadlift	10	3	3	4	4	45	30	45	30
2A	Dumbbell Push Press	10	3	3	4	4	45	30	45	30
2B	Kneeling Overhand-Grip Lat Pulldown	10	3	3	4	4	45	30	45	30
3	Side Bridge	60 sec	2	2	2	2	60	60	60	60

WORKOUT B

ORDER	EXERCISE	REPS	SETS				REST (IN SEC)			
			Week 1	Week 2	Week 3	Week 4	Week 1	Week 2	Week 3	Week 4
1A	Dumbbell Lunge	10	3	3	4	4	45	30	45	30
1B	Scaption + Shrug	10	3	3	4	4	45	30	45	30
2A	Swiss-Ball Hip Extension and Leg Curl	10	3	3	4	4	45	30	45	30
2B	Dumbbell Bench Press	10	3	3	4	4	45	30	45	30
3	Swiss-Ball Jackknife	10–15	2	2	2	2	60	60	60	60

PHASE 3: WEEKS 9 THROUGH 12

WORKOUT A

ORDER	EXERCISE	REPS	SETS				REST (IN SEC)			
			Week 1	Week 2	Week 3	Week 4	Week 1	Week 2	Week 3	Week 4
1	Front Squat	6	4	4	4	4	90	90	90	90
2A	Single-Arm Dumbbell Row	6	4	4	4	4	60	60	45	45
2B	Incline Dumbbell Bench Press	6	4	4	4	4	60	60	45	45
3	Chinup (or Negative Chinup)	6	4	4	4	4	90	90	90	90

WORKOUT B

ORDER	EXERCISE	REPS	SETS				REST (IN SEC)			
			Week 1	Week 2	Week 3	Week 4	Week 1	Week 2	Week 3	Week 4
1	Ipsilateral Back Lunge	12	3	3	3	3	60	60	45	45
2A	Leg Lowering Drill	12	3	3	3	3	45	45	30	30
2B	Incline Lower Trap Raise	12	3	3	3	3	45	45	30	30
3A	Pushup + Row	10	3	3	3	3	45	45	30	30
3B	Hip-Thigh Extension	12	3	3	3	3	45	45	30	30

THE ADVANCED WORKOUT

PHASE 1: WEEKS 1 THROUGH 4

WORKOUT A

ORDER	EXERCISE	REPS	SETS				REST (IN SEC)			
			Week 1	Week 2	Week 3	Week 4	Week 1	Week 2	Week 3	Week 4
1	Bulgarian Split Squat	8	3	3	3	3	90	90	90	90
2A	Barbell Bent-Over Row	8	3	3	3	3	60	60	60	60
2B	Dumbbell Bench Press	8	3	3	3	3	60	60	60	60
3A	Plank	60 sec	3	3	3	3	60	60	60	60
3B	Pullup (or Lat Pulldown)	8	3	3	3	3	60	60	60	60

WORKOUT B

ORDER	EXERCISE	REPS	SETS				REST (IN SEC)			
			Week 1	Week 2	Week 3	Week 4	Week 1	Week 2	Week 3	Week 4
1A	Goblet Squat	20	2	2	2	2	30	30	30	30
1B	V-Grip Seated Row	20	2	2	2	2	30	30	30	30
2A	Hip Extension	20	2	2	2	2	30	30	30	30
2B	Pushup	20	2	2	2	2	30	30	30	30
3A	Lat Pulldown	20	2	2	2	2	30	30	30	30
3B	Neutral-Grip Shoulder Press	20	2	2	2	2	30	30	30	30
4	Swiss-Ball Jackknife	15–20	2	2	2	2	45	45	45	45

WORKOUT C

ORDER	EXERCISE	REPS	SETS				REST (IN SEC)			
			Week 1	Week 2	Week 3	Week 4	Week 1	Week 2	Week 3	Week 4
1A	Walking Lunge	12	3	3	3	3	45	45	45	45
1B	Inverted Row	12	3	3	3	3	45	45	45	45
2A	Swiss-Ball Hip Extension and Leg Curl	12	3	3	3	3	45	45	45	45
2B	Dumbbell Bench Press	12	3	3	3	3	45	45	45	45
3A	Kneeling Reverse Cable Woodchop	12	2	2	2	2	45	45	45	45
3B	Pullup (or Lat Pulldown)	12	2	2	2	2	45	45	45	45

PHASE 2: WEEKS 5 THROUGH 8

WORKOUT A

ORDER	EXERCISE	REPS	SETS				REST (IN SEC)			
			Week 1	Week 2	Week 3	Week 4	Week 1	Week 2	Week 3	Week 4
1	Wide-Grip Deadlift	5	4	4	5	5	90	90	90	90
2A	Incline Dumbbell Bench Press	5	4	4	5	5	60	60	60	60
2B	Seated Row	5	4	4	5	5	60	60	60	60
3A	Chinup	5	4	4	5	5	60	60	60	60
3B	Incline Reverse Crunch	5	4	4	5	5	60	60	60	60

WORKOUT B

ORDER	EXERCISE	REPS	SETS				REST (IN SEC)			
			Week 1	Week 2	Week 3	Week 4	Week 1	Week 2	Week 3	Week 4
1	Contralateral Stepup	15	2	2	2	2	60	60	60	60
2A	Incline Dumbbell Bench Press	15	2	2	2	2	30	30	30	30
2B	Seated Row	15	2	2	2	2	30	30	30	30
3A	Kneeling Underhand-Grip Lat Pulldown	15	2	2	2	2	30	30	30	30
3B	Leg Lowering Drill	15	2	2	2	2	30	30	30	30

WORKOUT C

ORDER	EXERCISE	REPS	SETS				REST (IN SEC)			
			Week 1	Week 2	Week 3	Week 4	Week 1	Week 2	Week 3	Week 4
1	Wide-Grip Deadlift	10	3	3	3	3	75	75	75	75
2A	Incline Dumbbell Bench Press	10	3	3	3	3	45	45	45	45
2B	Seated Row	10	3	3	3	3	45	45	45	45
3A	Chinup	10	3	3	3	3	45	45	45	45
3B	Scaption + Shrug	10	3	3	3	3	45	45	45	45

PHASE 3: WEEKS 9 THROUGH 12
WORKOUT A

ORDER	EXERCISE	REPS	SETS				REST (IN SEC)			
			Week 1	Week 2	Week 3	Week 4	Week 1	Week 2	Week 3	Week 4
1	Barbell Squat	3	5	5	5	5	90	90	90	90
2A	Barbell Bent-Over Row	3	5	5	5	5	60	60	60	60
2B	Dumbbell Bench Press	3	5	5	5	5	60	60	60	60
3A	Good Morning	3	5	5	5	5	60	60	60	60
3B	Pullup	3	5	5	5	5	60	60	60	60

WORKOUT B

ORDER	EXERCISE	REPS	SETS				REST (IN SEC)			
			Week 1	Week 2	Week 3	Week 4	Week 1	Week 2	Week 3	Week 4
1	Thrusters	12	2	2	2	2	45	45	45	45
2A	Barbell Bent-Over Row	12	2	2	2	2	30	30	30	30
2B	Dumbbell Bench Press	12	2	2	2	2	30	30	30	30
3A	Back Extension	12	2	2	2	2	30	30	30	30
3B	Swiss-Ball Jackknife	12	2	2	2	2	30	30	30	30

WORKOUT C

ORDER	EXERCISE	REPS	SETS				REST (IN SEC)			
			Week 1	Week 2	Week 3	Week 4	Week 1	Week 2	Week 3	Week 4
1	Barbell Squat	8	3	3	3	3	60	60	60	60
2A	Barbell Bent-Over Row	8	3	3	3	3	45	45	45	45
2B	Dumbbell Bench Press	8	3	3	3	3	45	45	45	45
3A	Good Morning	8	3	3	3	3	45	45	45	45
3B	Chinup	8	3	3	3	3	45	45	45	45
4	Kneeling Reverse Cable Woodchop	8	3	3	3	3	60	60	60	60

BACK EXTENSION
Movement pattern: **Hip-Dominant**

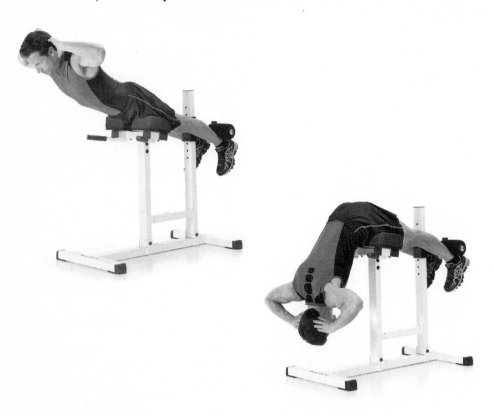

HOW TO DO IT:

1. Position yourself in the back-extension station and hook your feet under the leg anchors. Place your hands behind your head and lower your upper body, allowing your lower back to round, until it is just short of being perpendicular to the floor.

2. Raise your torso until it's in line with your lower body. At this point you should have a slight arch in your back and your shoulder blades should be pulled together in back.

3. Pause for 1 second, then take 3 seconds to lower your torso back to the starting position.

POINTERS: If this is too easy, you can either hold a weight plate across your chest, perform the exercise with only one foot hooked under the anchors (your other foot can rest on top), or do both. Keep in mind, performing the single-leg version will increase your workout time slightly because you'll have to train each leg separately.

BARBELL BENT-OVER ROW
Movement pattern: **Horizontal Pull**

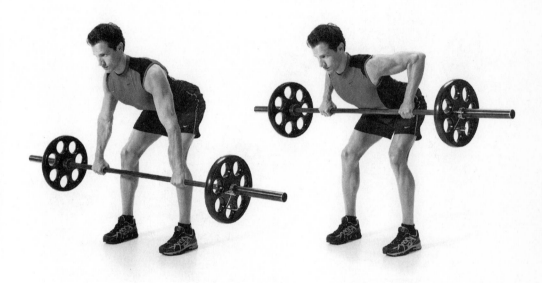

HOW TO DO IT:

1. Grab a barbell with an overhand grip that's just beyond shoulder width, and hold it at arm's length. Stand with your feet shoulder width apart and knees slightly bent. Bend at the hips, keeping your lower back flat, and lower your torso until it's almost parallel to the floor. Let the bar hang straight down from your shoulders.

2. Pull the bar up to your torso.

3. Pause for 1 second, then take 3 seconds to lower the bar back to the starting position.

POINTER: Even with detailed instructions, this exercise is frequently executed with improper form. That's because many people don't understand how to keep their lower back "flat." They allow it to round, which can lead to injury (read: slipped disk). To avoid that mistake, stand up tall when you first pick up the barbell—with your lower back naturally arched—and think of your upper body as being rigid. Then, instead of simply bending over, push your hips backward as far as possible while trying to keep your entire upper body rigid as you lower it down to parallel. If you look in a mirror and your lower back isn't flat, you're doing it wrong.

BARBELL SQUAT
Movement pattern: **Quadriceps-Dominant**

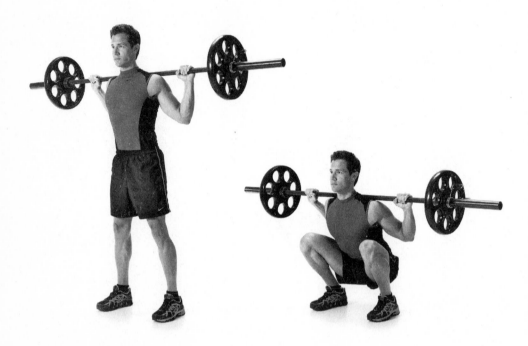

HOW TO DO IT:

1. Hold a bar across your upper back with an overhand grip, your feet set shoulder width apart and your shoulders pulled back. The bar should sit comfortably on the shelf created by your shoulder blades.

2. Lift the bar off the rack and step back. Set your feet shoulder width apart, knees slightly bent, back straight, eyes focused straight ahead.

3. Initiate the movement by pushing your hips backward, then bend your knees and take 3 seconds to lower your body as far as possible. (The deeper you squat, the better.)

4. Pause for 1 second, then push your body back to the starting position.

POINTER: If you can't lower your body until your upper thighs are at least parallel to the floor, widen your stance and point your toes outward a little more. Then hold the deepest position possible for a two-count each repetition. Try to lower your body a little farther with each subsequent workout. As your flexibility improves, narrow your stance and decrease the angle that your toes point out.

BULGARIAN SPLIT SQUAT
Movement pattern: **Quadriceps-Dominant**

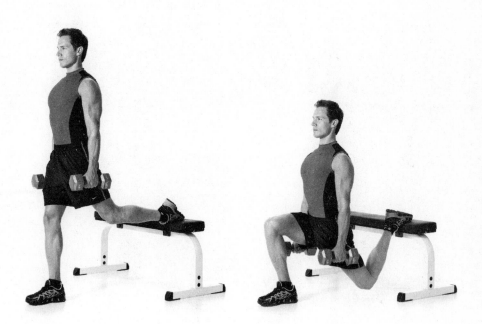

HOW TO DO IT:

1. Grab a pair of dumbbells and stand 2 to 3 feet in front of a bench. Place your left foot behind you on the bench so that only your instep is resting on it. Hold the dumbbells at arm's length next to your sides.

2. Take 3 seconds to lower your body until your front knee is bent 90 degrees and your rear knee nearly touches the floor. Your front lower leg should be perpendicular to the floor and your torso should remain upright.

3. Pause for 1 second, then push yourself back to the starting position as quickly as you can. Finish all of your repetitions, then repeat the lift, this time with your right foot resting on the bench while your left leg performs the work.

POINTER: To keep your torso upright throughout the lift, start by standing up tall in the split squat position. Then, as you lower your body, remind yourself that your upper body should be perpendicular to the floor, and moving up and down in a straight line.

CHINUP
Movement pattern: **Vertical Pull**

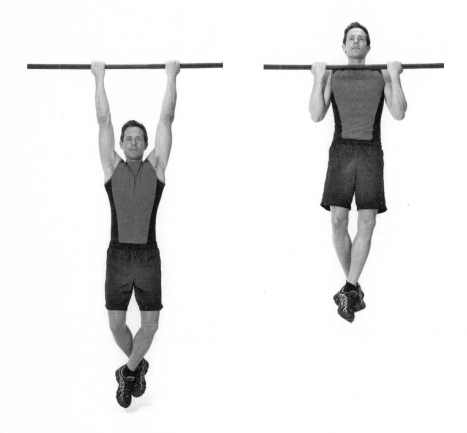

HOW TO DO IT:

1. Grab the chinup bar with a shoulder-width, underhand grip, cross your ankles behind you, and hang.

2. Pull yourself up as high as you can.

3. Pause for 1 second, then take 3 seconds to lower your body to the starting position.

POINTER: Imagine that you're pulling the bar to your chest, instead of your chest to the bar.

CHINUP (NEGATIVE)
Movement pattern: **Vertical Pull**

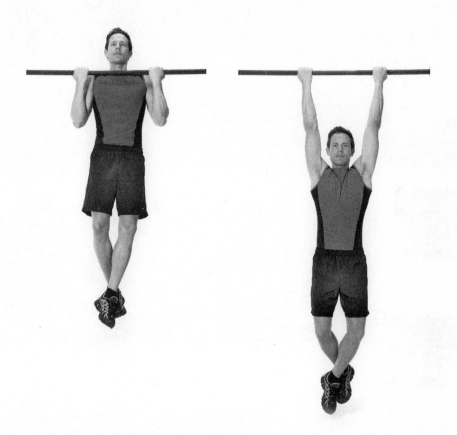

HOW TO DO IT:

1. Set a bench under a chinup bar. You'll use the bench to help you reach the bars. Step up on the bench and grasp the bar using an underhand grip.

2. From the bench, jump up so that your chest is next to your hands, then cross your feet behind you.

3. Try to take 5 seconds to lower your body until your arms are straight. If that's too hard, lower yourself as slowly as you can.

4. Jump up to the starting position and repeat.

POINTER: Try to lower your body at the same rate of speed from top to bottom. If you notice that you speed up at a specific point, make a mental note. Then, on your next set, pause for a second or two just above that point as you lower your body.

CONTRALATERAL STEPUP
Movement pattern: Hip-Dominant with Vertical Press

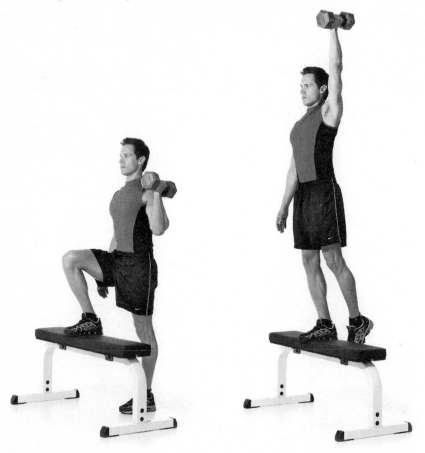

HOW TO DO IT:

1. Grab a dumbbell and hold it in your left hand, just outside your shoulder, your palm facing your body. Place your right foot on a bench, box, or step that's about knee height.

2. Push down with your right heel, and step up onto the bench as you push the dumbbell straight above your left shoulder. (Your left foot should be hanging off the bench.)

3. Lower your left foot back to the floor, and repeat until you've completed all of your repetitions. Then switch legs and arms, and do the same number of reps with your left foot on the bench, while pressing the weight with your right arm.

POINTER: Don't bother trying to lower your body slowly on this exercise. Simply perform the lifting portion of the movement in a fast, but controlled manner, then step down at a natural speed.

DUMBBELL BENCH PRESS
Movement pattern: **Horizontal Press**

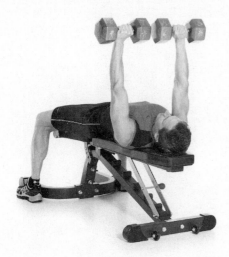

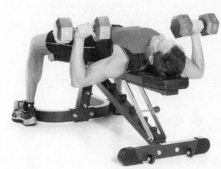

HOW TO DO IT:

1. Grab a pair of dumbbells and lie on your back on a flat bench, holding the dumbbells over your chest, nearly touching each other.

2. Take 3 seconds to lower the dumbbells to the sides of your chest, pause for 1 second, then press them back up to the starting position.

POINTER: When you press the dumbbells up, don't let them clang together. Some experts argue that it momentarily releases the tension on your muscles, reducing the exercise's effectiveness. We just think it's annoying.

DUMBBELL LUNGE
Movement pattern: **Quadriceps-Dominant**

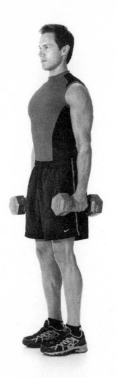
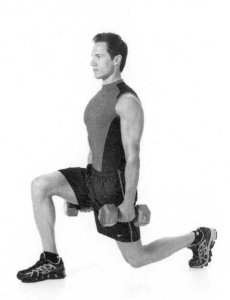

HOW TO DO IT:

1. Grab a pair of dumbbells and hold them at your sides. Stand with your feet hip width apart.

2. Step forward with your right leg, and take 2 seconds to lower your body until your front knee is bent 90 degrees and your rear knee nearly touches the floor. Your front lower leg should be perpendicular to the floor and your torso should remain upright.

3. Pause momentarily, then push yourself back up to the starting position as quickly as you can. Finish all of your repetitions, then repeat the lift, this time stepping forward with your left leg.

POINTER: To make the exercise harder without the use of heavier dumbbells, you can perform a "box" lunge by placing a 6-inch step or box in front of you. Simply step forward onto the box, and then lower your body. This increases your range of motion, which works more muscle.

DUMBBELL PULLOVER
Movement pattern: **Vertical Pull**

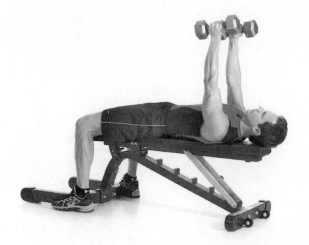

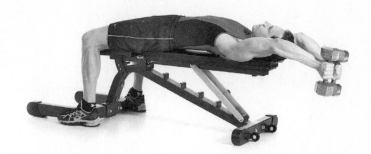

HOW TO DO IT:

1. Grab a pair of dumbbells and lie on your back on a flat bench with the weights straight over your chest and a little less than shoulder width apart. Your palms are turned toward each other, and your elbows are bent slightly.

2. Without changing the bend in your elbows, take 3 seconds to lower the dumbbells back beyond your head until your arms are in line with your body.

3. Pause for 1 second, then lift the weights back to the starting position.

POINTER: Try to keep the dumbbells even with each other as you lower and raise them.

DUMBBELL PUSH PRESS
Movement pattern: **Vertical Press with Quadriceps-Dominant**

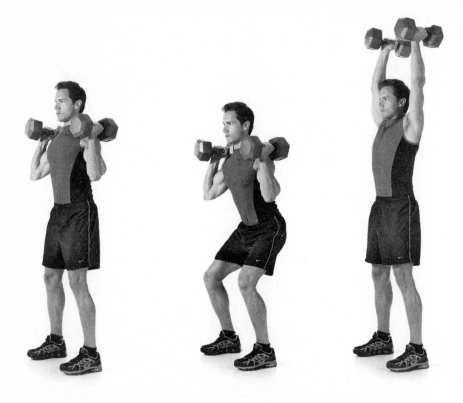

HOW TO DO IT:

1. Stand holding a pair of dumbbells just outside of your shoulders, your arms bent and palms facing each other. Your feet should be shoulder width apart and knees slightly bent.

2. Dip your knees slightly and push up with your legs as you press the dumbbells straight above each shoulder.

3. Take 3 seconds to lower the dumbbells back to the starting position, pause momentarily, then repeat.

POINTER: Make sure to allow your legs to help drive the dumbbells above your head. This is a powerful all-in-one movement that will allow you to use heavier dumbbells than a standard dumbbell shoulder press.

DUMBBELL STEPUP
Movement pattern: Hip-Dominant

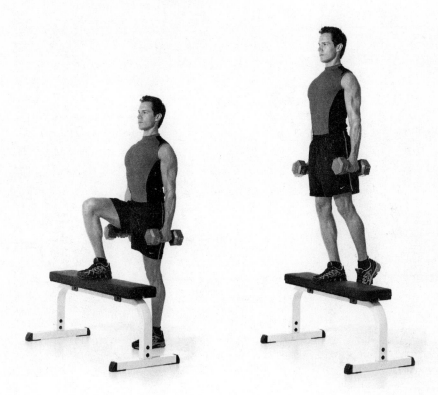

HOW TO DO IT:

1. Grab a pair of dumbbells and hold them at arm's length at your sides. Stand in front of a bench or step, and place your right foot firmly on the bench. The bench should be high enough so that your knee is bent 90 degrees.

2. Press your right heel into the bench and push your body up until your right leg is straight and you're standing on one leg on the bench, with your left foot hanging off the bench.

3. Lower your body until your left foot touches the floor. That's 1 repetition.

4. Once you've completed all of the prescribed repetitions with your right leg, repeat the exercise with your left leg.

POINTER: Don't bother trying to lower your body slowly on this exercise. Simply perform the lifting portion of the movement in a fast, but controlled manner, then step down at a natural speed.

FRONT SQUAT
Movement pattern: Quadriceps-Dominant

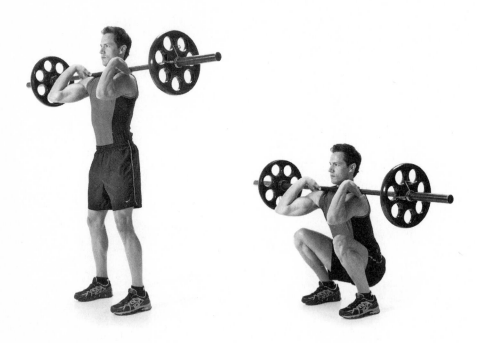

HOW TO DO IT:

1. Grab a bar with an overhand grip that's just beyond shoulder width, and hold it in front of your body, just above your shoulders. Raise your upper arms so they're parallel to the floor and let the bar roll back so it's resting on your fingers, not your palms. Set your feet shoulder width apart, and keep your back straight and your eyes focused straight ahead.

2. Without changing the position of your upper arms, take about 3 seconds to lower your body until your thighs are at least parallel to the floor. (The lower you can go, the better.)

3. Pause, then push yourself back up to the starting position.

POINTER: Keep your upper arms parallel to the floor for the entire lift. This ensures that your torso stays as upright as possible, for the most benefit and safety. Some guys aren't flexible enough to hold the bar this way. A second option is to cross your arms in front of you and allow the bar to rest on your shoulders. (You pick it up off the rack in this manner.) As another alternative, you can substitute the goblet squat on the opposite page.

GOBLET SQUAT
Movement pattern: Quadriceps-Dominant

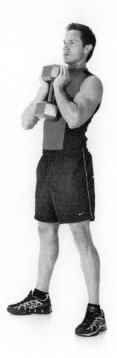

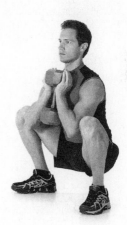

HOW TO DO IT:

1. Grab a dumbbell with both hands and hold it vertically in front of your chest. (Imagine that it's a heavy goblet.) Set your feet shoulder width apart.

2. Initiate the movement by pushing your hips backward, then bend your knees and take 3 seconds to lower your body as far as possible. (The deeper you squat, the better.) Keep your torso as upright as possible throughout the entire movement.

3. Pause, then push yourself back up to the starting position.

POINTER: Doing the goblet squat is one of the best ways to learn to squat naturally and safely. Don't be afraid to go as deep as possible. Research shows that the most unstable knee angle during the squat is when your knees are bent 90 degrees—a few inches above the point where your thighs are parallel to the floor. Plus, "full" squats strengthen your knee tendons and lead to balanced lower body development, unlike "shallow" squats, which can overdevelop your quadriceps and increase your risk for injury.

GOOD MORNING
Movement pattern: **Hip-Dominant**

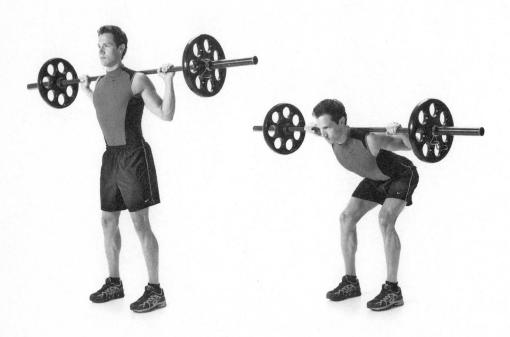

HOW TO DO IT:

1. Grab a barbell with an overhand grip and place it so that it rests comfortably across your upper back.

2. Take 3 seconds to lower the weight by bending forward at your hips, and lowering your torso as far as possible without allowing your lower back to round. Keep your head up and maintain the same angle of your knees throughout the lift.

3. Raise your upper body back to the starting position.

POINTER: Initiate the movement by first pushing your hips backward as far as possible.

HANGING LEG RAISE
Movement pattern: **Core**

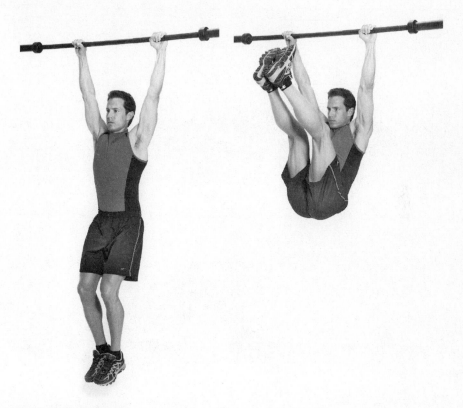

HOW TO DO IT:

1. Grab a chinup bar with an overhand, shoulder-width grip, and hang from the bar with your knees slightly bent and feet together. (If you have access to elbow supports—sling-like devices that hang from the bar—you may prefer to use those.)

2. Simultaneously bend your knees, raise your hips, and curl your lower back underneath you as you lift your thighs toward your chest.

3. Pause for 1 second when the fronts of your thighs reach your chest, then take 3 seconds to lower your legs back to the starting position.

POINTERS: Try to avoid these common mistakes:

1. Using momentum. Try staring straight ahead at all times—it will help your body stay upright.

2. Simply bending your knees and lifting your legs up. Instead, imagine scooping your hips up and forward.

3. Leaning backward. Your shoulders should remain in place or round forward slightly.

HIP EXTENSION
Movement pattern: Hip-Dominant

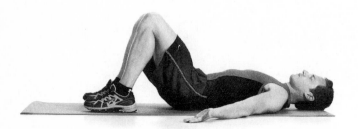

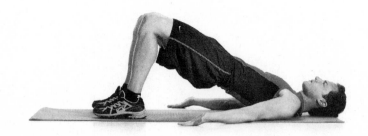

HOW TO DO IT:

1. Lie on your back on the floor with your knees bent and your feet flat on the floor. Place your arms out to your sides at a 45-degree angle, your palms facing up.

2. Raise your hips so your body forms a straight line from your shoulders to your knees.

3. Pause for 2 seconds, then take 2 seconds to lower your body back to the starting position.

POINTERS: If that's too easy, place a weight plate on your hips (you can secure it with your hands). To further increase the difficulty, perform the single-leg version of the exercise by pulling one knee to your chest for the entire movement. Finish all your repetitions, then switch legs and repeat.

HIP-THIGH EXTENSION
Movement pattern: **Hip-Dominant**

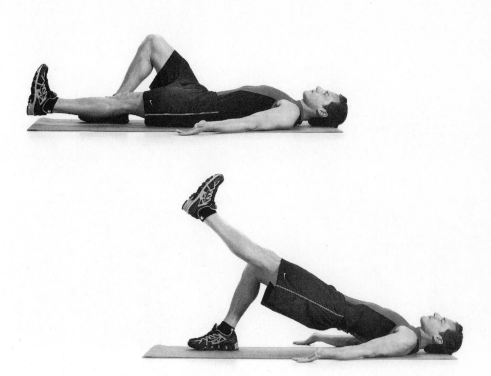

HOW TO DO IT:

1. Lie on your back on the floor with your right knee bent and your left leg straight. Place your arms out to your sides at a 45-degree angle, your palms facing up. Push your right heel into the floor until your entire body and your left leg are raised 1 inch off the floor. This is the starting position.

2. Raise your hips so your body forms a straight line from your shoulders to your right knee, and hold for 2 seconds.

3. Take 2 seconds to lower your body back to the starting position, pause for 1 second, and then repeat the movement.

4. After you've completed all of the prescribed repetitions, repeat with your left knee bent and your right leg straight.

POINTER: If that's too easy, cross your arms in front of your chest instead of placing them on the floor.

INCLINE DUMBBELL BENCH PRESS

Movement pattern: **Horizontal Press**

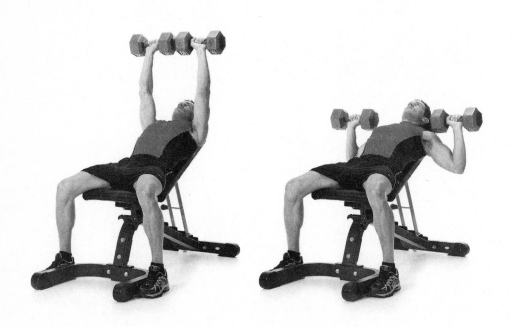

HOW TO DO IT:

1. Grab a pair of dumbbells and lie on your back on a bench set to a low incline (15 to 30 degrees). Lift the dumbbells so they're over your chin, and hold them so that they nearly touch, with your palms turned out (thumbs facing each other).

2. Take 3 seconds to lower the weights to your upper chest, pause for 1 second, then push them back up over your chin.

POINTER: The main function of your pectoralis major—your largest chest muscle—is to bring your upper arms across the front of your body. That's why you want to push the dumbbells not just up, but also toward each other during each repetition. (Think about this in the context of what happens to your upper arm.)

INCLINE LOWER TRAP RAISE
Movement pattern: **Vertical Press**

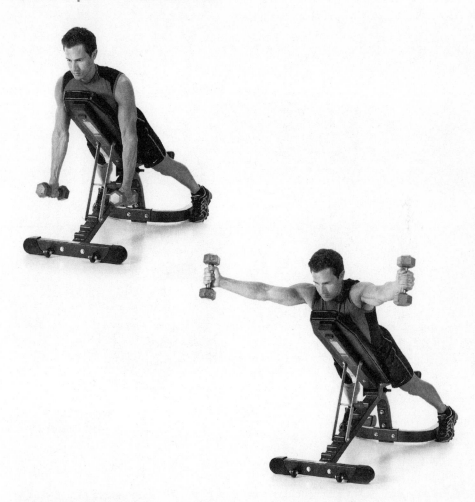

HOW TO DO IT:

1. Set an incline bench to a 30-degree angle. Grab a pair of dumbbells and lie with your chest against the pad. Let your arms hang straight down from your shoulders and turn your palms so they're facing each other. Keep your elbows slightly bent.

2. Without changing the bend in your elbows, raise your arms at a 30-degree angle to your body until they're in line with your torso.

3. Pause for 1 second, then take 3 seconds to lower the weights to the starting position.

POINTER: You know you're doing the exercise right if your arms form a "Y" when you raise them.

INCLINE REVERSE CRUNCH

Movement pattern: **Core**

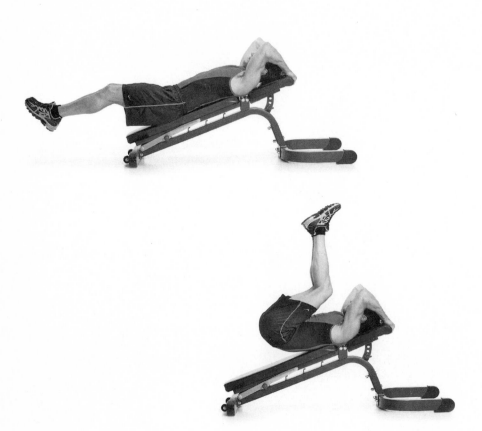

HOW TO DO IT:

1. Lie on a slant board with your hips lower than your head. Grab the bar behind your head for support, or simply grasp the sides of the board. Bend your knees slightly and hold your feet together.

2. Raise your knees to your chest by lifting your hips and crunching them inward, as if you were emptying a bucket of water that was resting on your pelvis.

3. Pause for 1 second, then take 3 seconds to lower your hips to the starting position.

POINTERS: If this exercise is too hard, perform the same exercise on the floor, with your arms out to your sides at a 90-degree angle, your palms facing up. If the exercise is too easy, you can hold a dumbbell between your feet as you perform the exercise, or substitute the hanging leg raise (page 179) instead.

INVERTED ROW
Movement pattern: **Horizontal Pull**

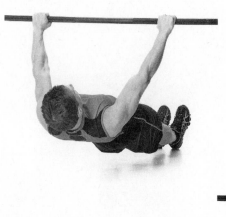

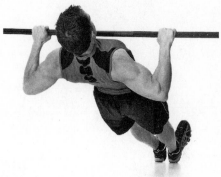

HOW TO DO IT:

1. Secure a bar 3 to 4 feet above the floor. Lie under the bar and grab it with a shoulder-width, overhand grip. Hang at arm's length from the bar with your body in a straight line from your ankles to your shoulders.

2. Keep your body rigid and pull your chest to the bar.

3. Pause, then lower yourself back to the starting position.

POINTERS: If this exercise is too hard, perform it with your knees bent 90 degrees and your feet placed flat on the floor. (This reduces the amount of your body weight you have to lift.) If the exercise is too easy, you can do the exercise with only one foot on the floor, or with both feet elevated—for instance, placed on a bench or a Swiss ball.

IPSILATERAL BACK LUNGE
Movement pattern: **Hip-Dominant with Vertical Press**

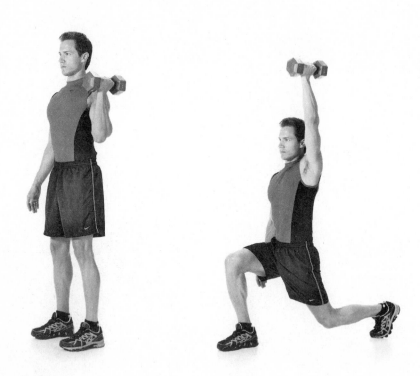

HOW TO DO IT:

1. Grab a dumbbell with your left hand, and hold it next to your left shoulder, your palm facing in, as if you were about to perform a neutral-grip shoulder press (page 192). Stand with your feet shoulder width apart.

2. Step backward with your left leg and lower your body until your front knee is bent 90 degrees and your rear knee nearly touches the floor. As you lower your body, simultaneously press the dumbbell straight above your shoulder until your arm is straight.

3. Lower the dumbbell as you push yourself back up to the starting position as quickly as you can. That's 1 repetition.

4. After you've completed all of the prescribed repetitions, switch arms and legs and repeat.

POINTER: Don't concern yourself with lowering your body at a particular speed; just perform it at a natural tempo that allows you to maintain control of your body and the weight at all times.

KNEELING OVERHAND-GRIP LAT PULLDOWN
Movement pattern: **Vertical Pull**

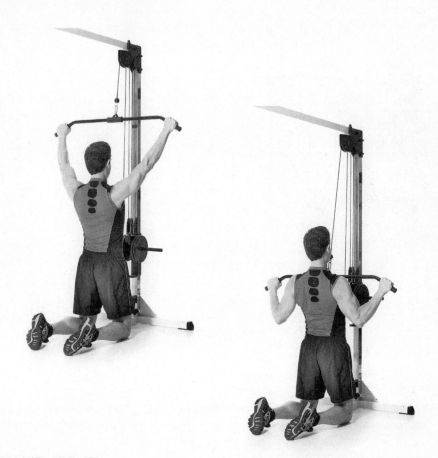

HOW TO DO IT:

1. Grab a lat pulldown bar with an overhand grip that's just beyond shoulder width. Then, instead of sitting in the machine, position yourself on your knees in front of it, your body forming a straight line from your shoulders to your knees. Your arms should be completely extended.

2. Pull the bar down to your chest.

3. Pause for 1 second, and then take 3 seconds to return to the starting position.

POINTERS: Don't lean back to pull the bar to your chest; your upper body should remain in nearly the same position from start to finish. Also, squeeze your shoulder blades together as you pull the bar down.

KNEELING REVERSE CABLE WOODCHOP

Movement pattern: Core

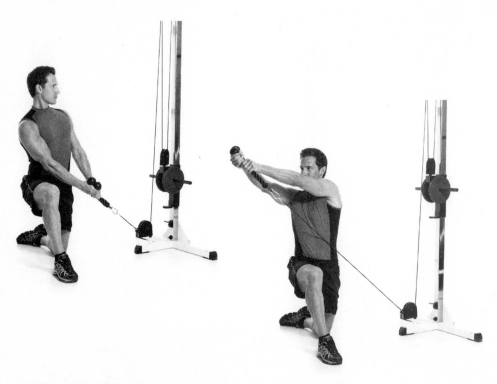

HOW TO DO IT:

1. Attach a rope handle to the low cable pulley of a cable station. Kneel down on your left knee next to the handle so that your left side faces the weight stack. Your right knee should be bent 90 degrees with your foot flat on the floor.

2. Rotate your body to grab the rope with both hands. Your shoulders will be turned toward the cable machine. Your arms should be nearly straight throughout the entire movement.

3. Pull the handle up and across your torso as you straighten your body and twist your shoulders to the right. Your left arm ends up in front of your face, and the handle is at the same height as your ear.

4. Pause, then slowly return to the starting position. Finish the repetitions on this side, then switch sides to complete the set.

POINTER: Focus on pulling the rope by rotating your torso, not by using your arms and shoulders.

KNEELING UNDERHAND-GRIP LAT PULLDOWN
Movement pattern: **Vertical Pull**

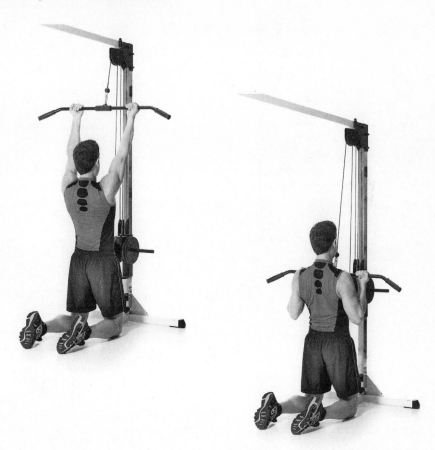

HOW TO DO IT:

1. Grab a lat pulldown bar with a shoulder-width, underhand grip. Then, instead of sitting in the machine, position yourself on your knees in front of it, your body forming a straight line from your shoulders to your knees. Your arms should be completely extended.

2. Pull the bar down to your chest.

3. Pause for 1 second, and then take 3 seconds to return to the starting position.

POINTERS: Don't lean back to pull the bar to your chest; your upper body should remain in nearly the same position from start to finish. Also, squeeze your shoulder blades together as you pull the bar down.

LAT PULLDOWN
Movement pattern: **Vertical Pull**

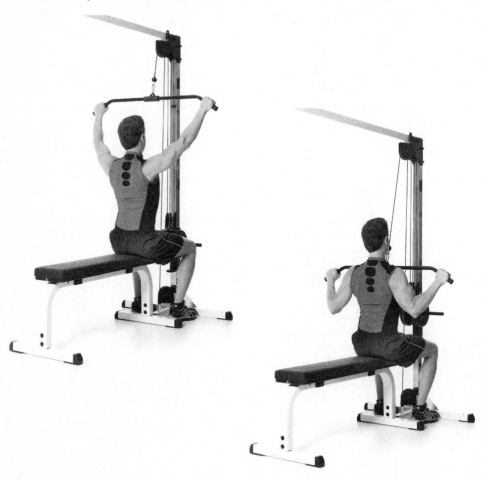

HOW TO DO IT:

1. Sit down in a lat pulldown machine and grab the bar with an overhand grip that's just beyond shoulder width. Your arms should be completely extended, and your knees secured under the leg anchors.

2. Pull the bar down to your chest.

3. Pause for 1 second, and then take 3 seconds to return to the starting position.

POINTERS: Don't lean back to pull the bar to your chest; your upper body should remain in nearly the same position from start to finish. Also, squeeze your shoulder blades together as you pull the bar down.

LEG LOWERING DRILL

Movement pattern: **Core**

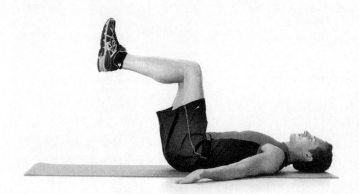

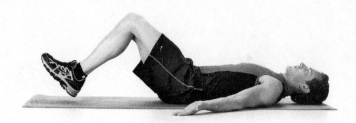

HOW TO DO IT:

1. Lie on your back on the floor, and raise your upper legs until they're perpendicular to the floor. Now bend your knees 90 degrees.

2. Without changing the angle of your knees, press your lower back flat into the floor and hold it there as you try to take 5 seconds to lower your feet to the floor.

3. Once your feet touch the floor, raise your legs back to the starting position, and repeat. Do 10 repetitions.

POINTER: If that's too easy, straighten your legs a little more. And keep doing so as it becomes easier, until you can perform the exercise with straight legs and without ever allowing your lower back to lose contact with the floor. If the exercise is too hard, determine where your back loses contact with the floor, and pause just above that point for a two-count each repetition.

NEUTRAL-GRIP SHOULDER PRESS
Movement pattern: **Vertical Press**

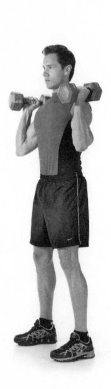
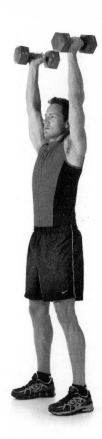

HOW TO DO IT:

1. Stand holding a pair of dumbbells just outside of your shoulders, with your arms bent and palms facing each other. Your feet should be shoulder width apart, your knees slightly bent.

2. Press the weights straight over your shoulders until your arms are straight.

3. Pause for 1 second, then take 3 seconds to lower the dumbbells back to the starting position.

POINTER: Make sure to push the dumbbells in a straight line, instead of pushing them up and toward each other as many people do, a habit that increases your risk for shoulder injuries.

PLANK
Movement pattern: **Core**

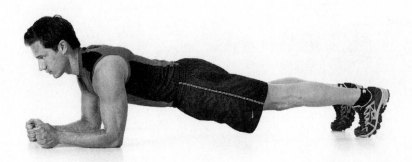

HOW TO DO IT:

1. Start to get into a pushup position, but bend your elbows and rest your weight on your forearms instead of your hands. Your body should form a straight line from your shoulders to your ankles.

2. Contract and brace your abdominals. (Imagine someone is about to punch you in the gut.)

3. Hold this position for 60 seconds.

POINTERS: If you can't hold the position for 60 seconds, hold for 5 to 10 seconds, rest for 5 seconds, and repeat as many times as needed to total 60 seconds. Each time you perform the exercise, try to hold each repetition a little longer, so that you reach your 60-second goal with fewer repetitions.

PRONE COBRA
Movement pattern: **Core**

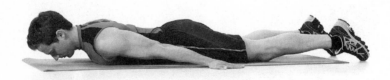

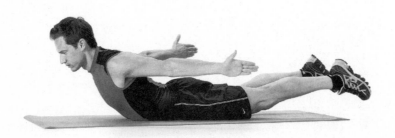

HOW TO DO IT:

1. Lie facedown on the floor with your legs straight, and your arms next to your sides, palms down.

2. Contract your glutes and the muscles of your lower back, and raise your chest and legs off the floor. Simultaneously rotate your arms so that your thumbs point toward the ceiling. At this time, the only part of your body that should be touching the floor is your hips.

3. Hold this position for 60 seconds.

POINTERS: If you can't hold the position for 60 seconds, hold for 5 to 10 seconds, rest for 5 seconds, and repeat as many times as needed to total 60 seconds. Each time you perform the exercise, try to hold each repetition a little longer, so that you reach your 60-second goal with fewer repetitions. If the exercise is too easy, you can hold dumbbells when you do it.

PULLUP
Movement pattern: **Vertical Pull**

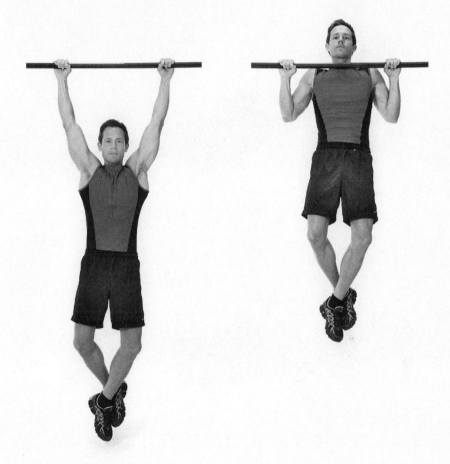

HOW TO DO IT:

1. Grab the pullup bar with an overhand grip that's just beyond shoulder width.

2. Cross your ankles behind you and hang.

3. Pull yourself up as high as you can.

4. Pause for 1 second, then take 3 seconds to lower your body to the starting position.

POINTER: Imagine you're pulling the bar to your chest, instead of your chest to the bar.

PUSHUP
Movement pattern: **Horizontal Press**

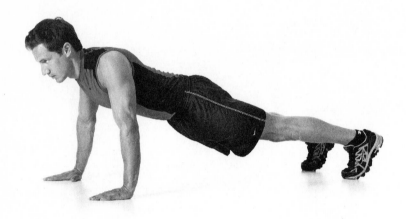

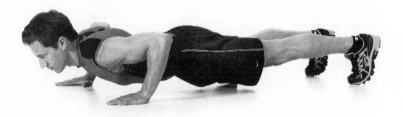

HOW TO DO IT:

1. Get into pushup position—your hands slightly wider and in line with your shoulders—with your body forming a straight line from your ankles to your shoulders. Your arms should be straight.

2. Take 3 seconds to lower your body as far as possible—your upper arms should drop lower than your elbows.

3. Pause for 1 second, then quickly push yourself back to the starting position.

POINTER: Keep your body rigid throughout the movement, particularly in regard to your hips. Your hips shouldn't sag at any time during the exercise.

PUSHUP + ROW
Movement pattern: Horizontal Press with Horizontal Pull

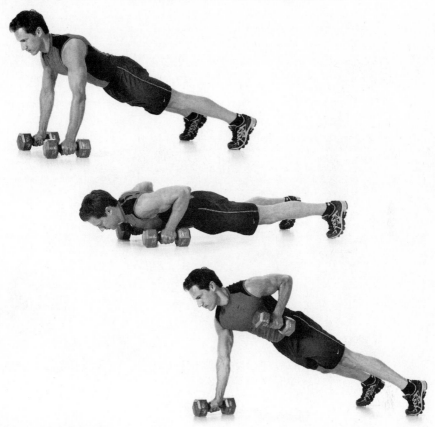

HOW TO DO IT:

1. Place hexagonal dumbbells just beyond shoulder width apart on the floor. Then, instead of placing your hands on the floor, get into pushup position by grasping the dumbbells. Your body should form a straight line from your ankles to your shoulders.

2. Take 3 seconds to lower your body as far as possible—your upper arms should drop lower than your elbows.

3. Pause for 1 second, then quickly push yourself up until your arms are straight.

4. Row the dumbbell in your left hand to the side of your chest, by pulling it upward and bending your arm. Your torso should not rotate. Pause momentarily, then lower the dumbbell back down quickly, and repeat the same movement on your right side. That's 1 repetition.

POINTER: Keep your body rigid throughout the movement, particularly in regard to your hips. Your hips shouldn't sag at any time during the exercise.

ROMANIAN DEADLIFT
Movement pattern: **Hip-Dominant**

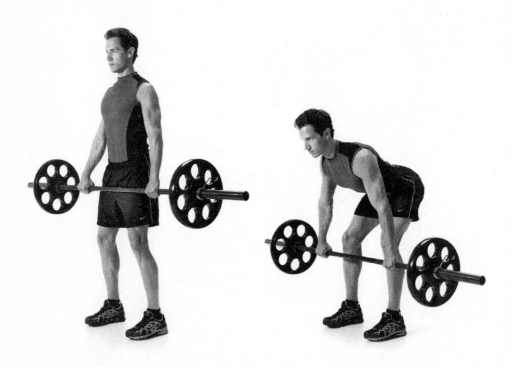

HOW TO DO IT:

1. Grab the bar with an overhand grip that's just beyond shoulder width. Stand holding the bar at arm's length and resting on the front of your thighs. Your feet are shoulder width apart and your knees slightly bent. Your eyes are focused straight ahead.

2. Slowly bend at the hips as you take 3 seconds to lower the bar as far as you can without allowing your lower back to round. Don't change the angle of your knees. Keep your head and chest up and your lower back flat or slightly arched.

3. Pause for 1 second, then lift your torso back to the starting position, keeping the bar as close to your body as possible.

POINTER: Start the movement by pushing your hips backward as far as you can.

SCAPTION + SHRUG
Movement pattern: **Vertical Pull**

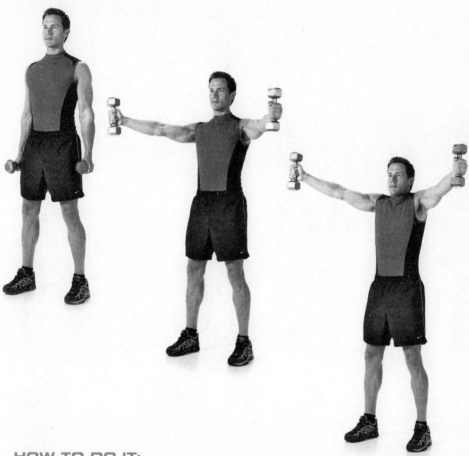

HOW TO DO IT:

1. Stand holding a pair of dumbbells with your feet shoulder width apart. Let the dumbbells hang at arm's length next to your sides, your palms facing each other and your elbows slightly bent.

2. Without changing the bend in your elbows, raise your arms at a 30-degree angle to your body (so that they form a "Y") until they're at shoulder level. Then shrug your shoulders upward.

3. Pause for 2 seconds, then take 2 seconds to lower the weight back to the starting position.

POINTER: To shrug, imagine that you're trying to touch your shoulders to your ears without moving any other parts of your body.

SEATED ROW
Movement pattern: **Horizontal Pull**

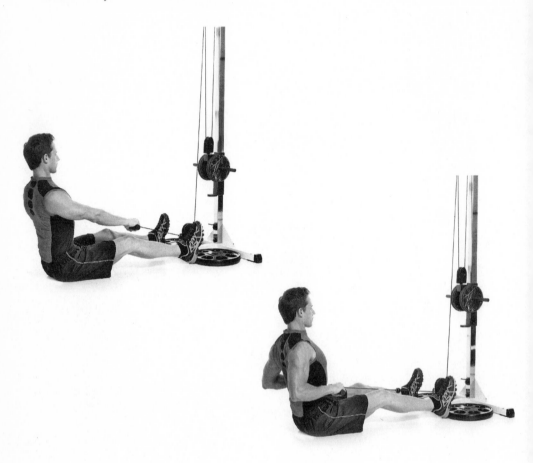

HOW TO DO IT:

1. Attach a straight bar to the cable and position yourself in the machine. Grab the bar with an overhand grip that's just beyond shoulder width. Sit up straight and pull your shoulders back.

2. Pull the bar to your abdomen by bending your arms and squeezing your shoulder blades together.

3. Pause for 2 seconds, then take 2 seconds to return to the starting position.

POINTER: Your torso should remain upright and motionless throughout the movement. So don't lean forward and back to perform the movement.

SEATED ROW TO NECK
Movement pattern: **Horizontal Pull**

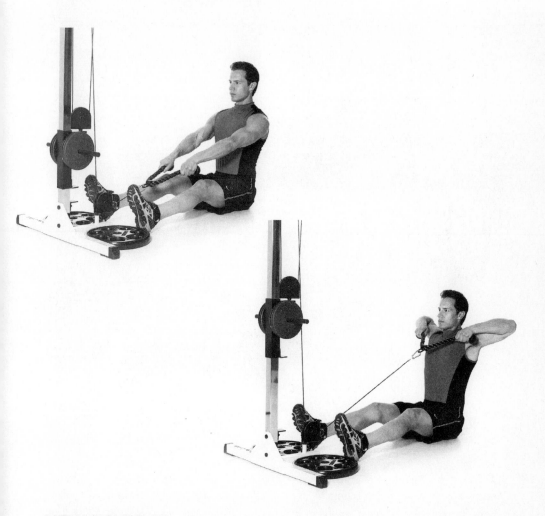

HOW TO DO IT:

1. Attach a rope handle to the cable and position yourself in the machine. Grab a rope in each hand, and sit up straight.

2. Pull the rope to your neck by bending your arms and squeezing your shoulder blades together.

3. Pause for 2 seconds, then take 2 seconds to return to the starting position.

POINTER: Your torso should remain upright and motionless throughout the movement. So don't lean forward and back to perform the movement.

SIDE BRIDGE
Movement pattern: **Core**

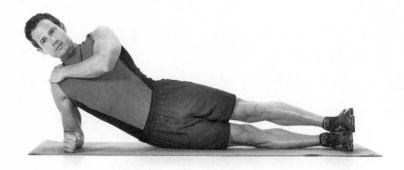

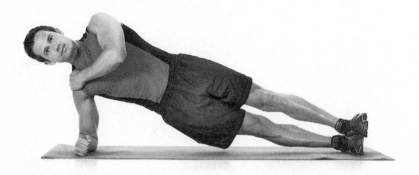

HOW TO DO IT:

1. Lie on your right side with your knees straight. Prop your upper body up on your right elbow and forearm, which should be directly below your right shoulder. Place your left hand on your right shoulder and raise your hips until your body forms a straight line from your ankles to your shoulders.

2. Contract and brace your abdominals. (Imagine someone is about to punch you in the gut.)

3. Hold this position for 60 seconds.

POINTERS: If you can't hold the position for 60 seconds, hold for 5 to 10 seconds, rest for 5 seconds, and repeat as many times as needed to total 60 seconds. Each time you perform the exercise, try to hold each repetition a little longer, so that you reach your 60-second goal with fewer repetitions.

SINGLE-ARM DUMBBELL ROW
Movement pattern: **Horizontal Pull**

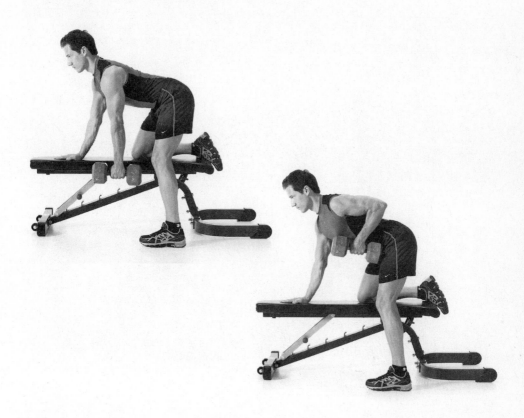

HOW TO DO IT:

1. Grab a dumbbell in your left hand and place your right hand and right knee on a flat bench. Keep your back flat and your upper body parallel to the floor. Let your left arm hang straight down at your side. Turn your palm so that it's facing your left leg.

2. Pull the dumbbell up to the side of your chest by bending your elbow and squeezing your shoulder blade toward the middle of your back. Keep your elbow close to your body.

3. Pause, then take 3 seconds to lower the dumbbell back to the starting position. After you've performed all of your repetitions with your left arm, immediately repeat the exercise with your right arm, placing your left arm and knee on the bench. Once complete, rest for the prescribed rest period.

POINTER: When you do the movement, imagine you're starting a lawn mower.

STATIC LUNGE
Movement pattern: **Quadriceps-Dominant**

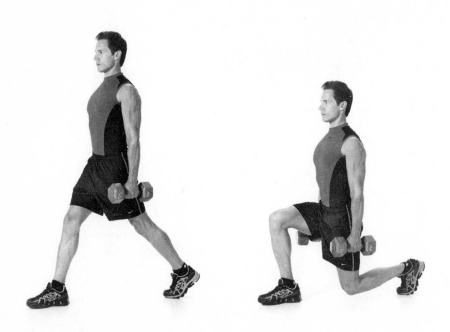

HOW TO DO IT:

1. Grab a pair of dumbbells and hold them at your sides. Stand in a staggered stance with your feet 2 to 3 feet apart, your right foot in front of your left.

2. Take 3 seconds to lower your body until your front knee is bent 90 degrees and your rear knee nearly touches the floor. Your front lower leg should be perpendicular to the floor and your torso should remain upright.

3. Pause for 1 second, then push yourself back up to the starting position as quickly as you can. Finish all of your repetitions, then repeat the exercise with your left foot in front of your right.

POINTER: Imagine that you're lowering your body straight down, not forward and down.

SWISS-BALL HIP EXTENSION AND LEG CURL

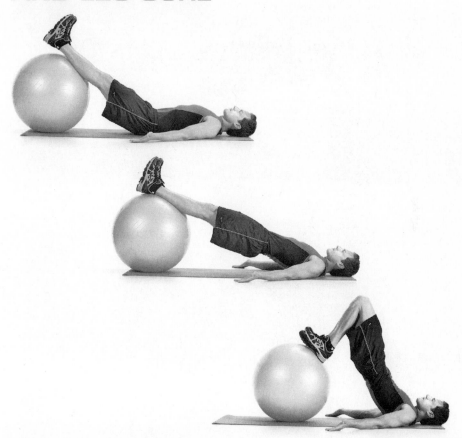

Movement pattern: **Hip-Dominant**

HOW TO DO IT:

1. Lie on your back on the floor and place your lower legs on a Swiss ball. Place your arms out to your sides at a 45-degree angle, your palms facing up.

2. Push your hips up so that your body forms a straight line from your shoulders to your ankles.

3. Without pausing, pull your heels toward you and roll the ball as close as possible to your butt.

4. Pause for 1 second, then reverse the motion by rolling the ball back until your body is in a straight line. Lower your hips back to the floor and repeat.

POINTER: Focus on keeping your hips in line with the rest of your body as you pull the ball toward you.

SWISS-BALL JACKKNIFE
Movement pattern: **Core**

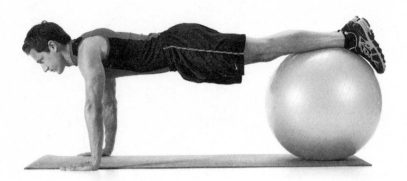

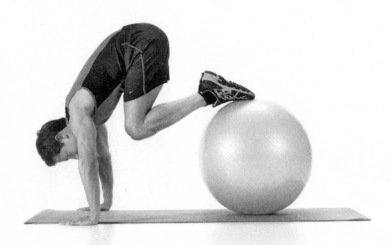

HOW TO DO IT:

1. Get into pushup position—your hands set slightly wider than and in line with your shoulders—but instead of placing your feet on the floor, rest your shins on a Swiss ball. With your arms straight and your back flat, your body should form a straight line from your shoulders to your ankles.

2. Roll the Swiss ball toward your chest by raising your hips and rounding your back as you pull the ball forward with your feet.

3. Pause, then return the ball to the starting position by lowering your hips and rolling it backward.

POINTER: Push your hips as high as you can as you roll the ball toward your chest.

THRUSTERS
Movement pattern: **Quadriceps-Dominant with Vertical Press**

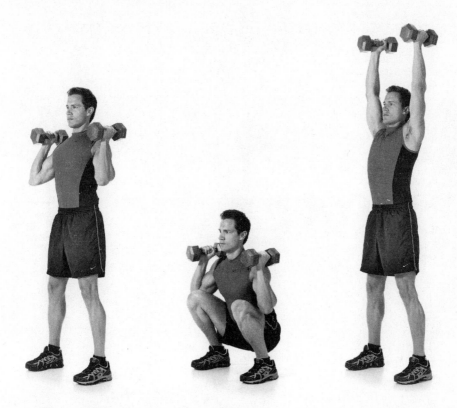

HOW TO DO IT:

1. Grab a pair of dumbbells and hold them next to your shoulders, your palms facing each other. Set your feet shoulder width apart, with your back straight and your eyes focused straight ahead.

2. Initiate the movement by pushing your hips backward, then bend your knees and take 3 seconds to lower your body as far as possible. (The deeper you squat, the better.)

3. Pause for 1 second, then push your body back up as you press the dumbbells directly over your shoulders until your arms are straight.

4. Lower the dumbbells back to the starting position, then repeat.

POINTER: Keep your torso as upright as possible throughout the movement.

V-GRIP SEATED ROW
Movement pattern: **Horizontal Pull**

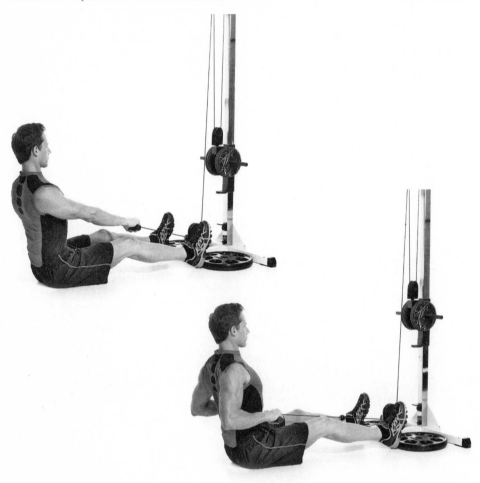

HOW TO DO IT:

1. Attach a V-grip handle to the cable and position yourself in the machine. (A straight bar is shown in the photo; you'll do the same movement but using the handle shaped like a V, so that your palms face each other when you grasp it.) Grab the handle with both hands and sit up straight.

2. Pull the handle to your abdomen by bending your arms and squeezing your shoulder blades together.

3. Pause for 2 seconds, then take 2 seconds to return to the starting position.

POINTER: Your torso should remain upright and motionless throughout the movement. So don't lean forward and back to perform the movement.

WALKING LUNGE
Movement pattern: **Quadriceps-Dominant**

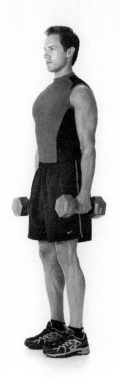 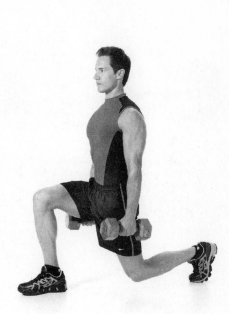

HOW TO DO IT:

1. Grab a pair of dumbbells and hold them at your sides. Stand with your feet hip width apart.

2. Step forward with your right leg, and take **2** seconds to lower your body until your front knee is bent 90 degrees and your rear knee nearly touches the floor. Your front lower leg should be perpendicular to the floor, and your torso should remain upright.

3. Pause momentarily, then push off your right leg and step forward with your left leg so that your body is in the starting position again but a full lunge-step ahead of where you began. (That is, you'll be walking forward with each lunge.) Then repeat, lunging forward with your left leg. That's **1** repetition. Continue to alternate legs until you complete the prescribed number of repetitions.

POINTER: If you're limited on space, simply turn around once you have no room to lunge forward and then continue your set.

WIDE-GRIP DEADLIFT
Movement pattern: **Hip-Dominant**

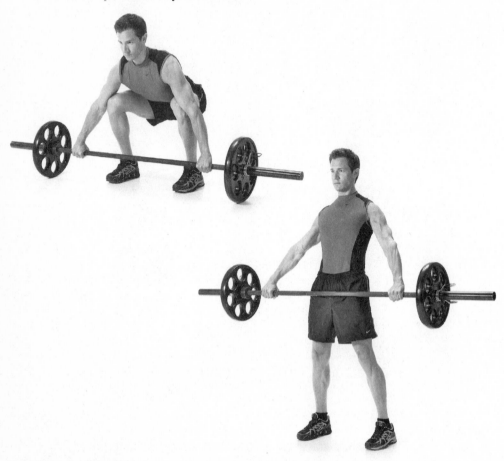

HOW TO DO IT:

1. Load the barbell and roll it against your shins. Grab the bar with an overhand grip, your hands about twice shoulder width. Squat down, focus your eyes straight ahead, and pull your shoulders back. Your arms should be straight, and your lower back flat, not rounded.

2. Without allowing your lower back to round, stand up with the barbell, thrusting your hips forward.

3. Pause momentarily, then take 3 seconds to reverse the movement and lower the bar to the floor, keeping it as close to your body as possible.

POINTER: Focus on keeping your lower back flat throughout the entire movement. If you're not able to, the weight is too heavy for you.

WIDE-GRIP SEATED ROW
Movement pattern: **Horizontal Pull**

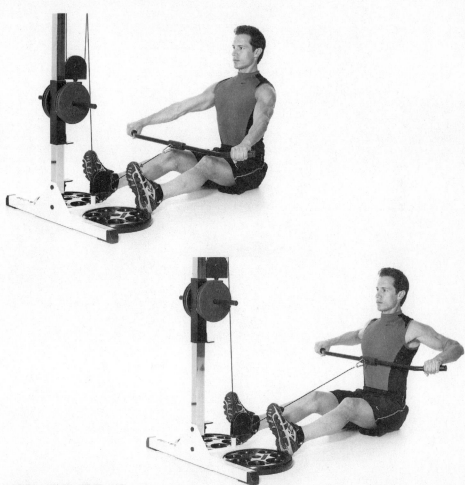

HOW TO DO IT:

1. Attach a lat pulldown bar to the cable and position yourself in the machine. Grab the bar with an overhand grip that's just beyond shoulder width. Sit up straight and pull your shoulders back.

2. Pull the bar to your chest by bending your arms and squeezing your shoulder blades together.

3. Pause for 2 seconds, then take 2 seconds to return to the starting position.

POINTER: Your torso should remain upright and motionless throughout the movement. So don't lean forward and back to perform the movement.

PART V:
YOUR HEALTH

CHAPTER 12

LOOK BETTER, LIVE LONGER

Take your age. Now add 20 years. That's the effect that an oversized gut has on your health, according to a UCLA study. Which means that the quest for a lean midsection, through diet and exercise, isn't a shallow pursuit; it's the only *natural* way to increase your lifespan. Or at the very least, ensure that you *live* up to your full potential.

It's important to understand that belly fat isn't just lifeless tissue that only serves to make you cringe at the idea of taking your shirt off in public. Fat can actually act like an endocrine organ, secreting numerous hormone and hormone-like substances—called adipokines—into your bloodstream. In fact, scientists have identified more than 50 different kinds of adipokines, many of which are harmful. One is called *resistin,* a hormone that leads to high blood sugar, an independent risk factor for heart disease and diabetes. There's also *angiotensinogen,* a compound that raises blood pressure, and *interleukin-6,* a chemical that causes arterial inflammation. What's more, a landmark discovery was the finding that an adipokine called *retinol-binding protein 4* (RBP4) caused insulin resistance and diabetes. While drug companies are now racing to find methods to lower RBP4, we showed in a recent study that a low-carbohydrate diet reduced levels by more than 20 percent. In the same study, we found that a low-fat, high-carb diet increased RBP4.

Your body actually houses two main types of fat: subcutaneous and visceral. Although displeasing to the eye, subcutaneous fat, which is located just under the skin and in front of your abdominal muscles, appears to be the less harmful of the two. This is the fat that you can pinch—or the kind that jiggles. Visceral fat, on the other hand, lurks behind your abdominal muscles, and surrounds your internal organs. Even though it's the less aesthetically harmful of the two fats (it doesn't jiggle, although it does push your belly out), scientists have concluded it's far more active than subcutaneous fat, making it markedly more dangerous to your health. You might liken the difference between subcutaneous and visceral fat to that of a dormant volcano compared to one that's constantly erupting. The latter is spewing out nasty stuff all the time; the other—subcutaneous fat—is just part of the landscape.

Worse, unlike other endocrine organs such as your pancreas, fat has the unique ability to expand. This potential is especially problematic where visceral fat is concerned. The larger visceral fat cells grow, the more dysfunctional—and dangerous—they become.

If your belly is bulging with visceral fat, it's likely that you are, or will soon be, *insulin resistant.* As discussed earlier, insulin is a hormone whose primary function is moving glucose out of your bloodstream and into your cells. This process helps you maintain normal, healthy blood sugar levels. Problems arise, however, when, often due to weight gain, your cells start to become resistant to the effects of insulin (it knocks, no one answers). As a result, more insulin is required to dispose of the same amount of glucose (the knock becomes a loud banging). This condition, called insulin resistance, is the first stage in type 2 diabetes. (Once you develop diabetes, you'll be able to predict the future: There's an 80 percent chance your cause of death will be heart disease.) If you think this doesn't apply to you, there's nearly a one in two chance you're wrong. Currently, it's estimated that *at least* 43 percent of American men are insulin resistant. That number is staggering, especially when you consider it includes all men—even very lean ones—making the prevalence of the condition even greater among those with the high-risk waistlines. The bottom line: If your gut is growing larger, you're probably on your way toward insulin resistance—even if your belly jiggles, since there's probably plenty of visceral fat underneath it.

What's more, without treatment, insulin resistance worsens over time. As a result, your pancreas has to pump out enormous amounts of insulin to force glucose into your cells (hey, let's use a sledgehammer!). This is called hyper-insulinemia. As this dysfunction intensifies, and even large amounts of insulin can no longer maintain glucose levels, you enter into a period where blood sugar is moderately elevated at all times—a condition known as *impaired glucose tolerance.* Over one-third of adults in the United States suffer from glucose intolerance according to a recent National Institutes of Health study. Eventually, your pancreas has trouble keeping up, leaving you with chronic high blood sugar, the defining marker of diabetes and the root cause of the calamities—heart disease, kidney failure, blindness, gangrene—that arise from it. Alas, it only gets worse from there: If the resistance continues to mount, some of the insulin-producing beta cells inside your pancreas can "burn out" and stop working altogether. Once this happens, you're looking at a lifetime of daily insulin injections.

Keep in mind, insulin resistance progresses over time. Long before being diagnosed with diabetes, other symptoms appear, all of which seem to be related. So much so, in fact, that some scientists have termed it *metabolic syndrome*. Metabolic syndrome describes a condition in which a person is inflicted with a cluster of heart disease risk factors. You are an unlucky qualifier if you have any three of the following five markers: a 40-inch (or greater) waist, high triglycerides (a type of fat in your bloodstream), high blood sugar, low HDL (good) cholesterol, and high blood pressure. This murderer's row of maladies is lethal. It increases the likelihood you'll develop diabetes by 500 percent, have a heart attack by 300 percent, and *die* of a heart attack by 200 percent. All of which is why the pharmaceutical industry has created drugs like rimonabant—branded under the name Acomplia—to treat the markers of metabolic syndrome, including obesity. These drugs, though, have limited success and are not without side effects.

Thankfully, there's a far more effective therapy than medication: low-carbohydrate diets. Research from our lab and many others has shown that simply restricting carbohydrates improves all of the markers of metabolic syndrome. In fact, the opposite approach—eating a low-fat, high-carb diet—will actually make metabolic syndrome worse unless you also lose weight and exercise more.

But unlike any other approach, low-carb diets decrease your risk of metabolic syndrome and its deadly consequences *even if you don't lose weight and exercise.* So from day one, you can put yourself at less risk when you follow the TNT Diet. Start shedding some pounds and hitting the gym, and you're going to be even better off. This is an important point because the conventional view is that low-carbohydrate diets improve metabolic markers only because people lose weight. The truth is that the low-carb approach directly improves metabolic syndrome because of the way it impacts your glycogen and insulin levels. Sure, weight loss generally does occur, and in fact, to a greater extent than low-fat diets in most studies. But again the point is that weight loss is not necessary to see metabolic improvement, whereas with low-fat diets it is.

In a recent study, we compared a low-carb, high-fat diet to a low-fat, high-carb diet for 12 weeks. We measured several markers of disease risk, including those of metabolic syndrome. The results were amazing. The low-carb approach far outperformed the low-fat diet. For example, the guys who

(continued on page 221)

The Truth about Low-Carb Diets

When you start a diet, everyone has an opinion on it—your co-workers, your buddy, even your 90-year-old grandmother. That's why it's important that you know all the facts. After all, we wouldn't want you to start doubting the TNT Diet due to a conversation with a misinformed relative. Throughout this chapter and this book, we've shown that unlike once thought, low-carb diets are fantastic for reducing your heart disease risk, and that eating fat doesn't make you fat. But here are three more low-carb myths that are still being perpetuated—on morning talk shows, in office break rooms, and at family get-togethers across America.

Myth 1: "Low-carb diets cause ketosis—and that's dangerous!"

When you reduce your carbohydrate intake significantly—typically to less than 50 to 75 grams a day—you enter a metabolic state known as *ketosis*. Ketosis is a term used to describe the *normal* process of using ketones for energy. Ketones aren't bad. They're actually a fat breakdown product. That is, whenever fat is burned, ketones are created. So they're always present in the body.

On a high-carb diet, your body uses glucose, the simplest form of carbohydrates, as its primary fuel. But when glucose isn't readily available to your body for energy—such as when you're in the Fat-Burning Time Zone—your body begins burning fat at an accelerated rate, producing more ketones. These ketones are really just storage units, holding the excess energy that's produced from the rapid breakdown of fat so that it can be later used as fuel. As ketone levels rise, your body's reliance on glucose decreases.

In the simplest terms, ketosis is just a shift from using carbohydrates (glucose) as the body's main energy source, to using fat (ketones). It's not a dangerous condition; it's simply your body adjusting to your diet so that it's using the most efficient form of fuel.

Unfortunately, many health professionals believe ketosis to be a dangerous metabolic condition. Why? Because over a hundred years ago, physicians discovered an overabundance of ketones in the urine of diabetics who were unable to control their disease. Naturally, the association of high levels of ketones with poorly controlled diabetes led to negative views of ketones. The high level of ketones in diabetics was given the name *diabetic hyperketoacidosis* (now known simply as *diabetic ketoacidosis).*

Diabetic ketoacidosis, which represents extremely high levels of ketones, is a life-threatening state that can occur in type 1 diabetics who aren't treating their condition appropriately. While diabetic ketoacidosis is serious, the mere presence of ketones is not. The point here is that sometimes a lot of something causes problems, but a little can be advantageous. Sort of like your heart beating 300 times a minute might be bad, but your heart beating 60 times a minute is ideal—and certainly better than not at all. Now consider: The ketone levels in people with diabetic ketoacidosis are 8 times higher than those following a low-carb diet.

Interestingly, ketones have many benefits. In fact, they may be the perfect fuel for dieters. Since ketones spare the use of carbohydrates for energy, they prevent the protein from your muscles from being broken down and converted to glucose. And that ensures that the calories you're burning are far more likely to be fat, compared to typical diets where muscle loss almost always accompanies fat loss. Ketones also suppress your appetite. Research shows that increased levels of a compound called beta-hydroxybutyrate—the primary ketone in the blood—act as a satiety signal, meaning it tells your brain that you're full.

Of course, the other knock on ketosis is that even if it burns fat faster, it deprives your brain of glucose, reducing your mental capacity. However, your brain only requires a small amount of glucose, which can be met through *gluconeogenesis,* the process of converting protein to glucose. Although not high in protein, by its nature a low-carb diet provides ample incoming protein. So there's plenty available for the small amount of glucose that your brain needs, without having to break down muscle. In addition, encouraging new research from National Institutes of Health scientist Richard Veech, MD, PhD, has found that ketones may help both your brain and heart run 25 percent more efficiently.

Myth 2: "Low-carb diets are bad for your kidneys!"

We hear this one a lot. The first flaw is that this claim is based on the assumption that low-carb diets are excessively high in protein, which some experts say forces your kidneys to work harder. (We'll address that point in a minute.) Unless you're consciously trying to down lots of protein by drinking several protein shakes a day, more than likely just 20 to 30 percent of your calories will come from protein. That's more than what the average American eats, but certainly not at a level that's going to strain healthy kidneys. In fact, most Americans probably don't eat enough protein. And of course, you need even more than the average person because you'll be hitting the weights hard 3 days a week. Research shows that guys who pump iron need almost twice as much protein as those who don't exercise. For reference, about a gram of protein each day per pound of lean body mass (your body weight minus the amount of body fat you have) seems to be about right—and certainly not excessive.

All that said, the idea that high-protein diets overstrain your kidneys seems to be perpetuated by people unfamiliar with the research. Read the scientific papers and you'll see that what's been found is that higher protein intake causes an increase in *glomerular filtration rate,* or GFR. Think of GFR as a measure of how much blood your kidneys are filtering per minute. This has been erroneously interpreted as an adverse effect when, in fact, it should be considered a normal physiologic adaptation to higher protein intakes. Consider an analogy with the heart: Exercise causes the heart to enlarge. Why? Because the heart muscles grow larger in order to push more blood throughout the body with less effort. Although an enlarged heart is also a consequence of heart disease, a bigger heart from exercise is not viewed as pathological, but rather, a positive physiological adaptation. It's a similar effect with protein and GFR. If you have kidney disease, you may have an elevated GFR. However, an elevated GFR doesn't mean that you have kidney disease—just like an enlarged heart from exercise doesn't mean that you have cardiovascular disease. Still, it's really a moot point when it comes to low-carb diets, such as the TNT Diet, which don't provide excessive amounts of protein anyway.

Myth 3: "Low-carb diets lead to bone loss!"

In contrast to the scientific evidence, another common criticism of diets low in carbohydrates, and again, high in protein, is bone loss. This concern seems to be based on a misunderstanding of basic metabolism. Critics claim that low-carbohydrate diets, and diets rich in animal protein, increase the acidity of your blood, which causes calcium to be leached from your bones. The theory is that because calcium is alkaline—the opposite of acidic—it's used by the body to buffer the higher acid levels, bringing blood pH levels back to normal. To support this notion, these critics cite evidence that higher protein intakes are associated with acute increases in the amount of calcium excreted in the urine. This, they say, is an indicator of calcium loss from the bones. Over time, this is suggested to cause actual bone loss.

However, this mechanism of bone loss is not substantiated by clinical data or long-term epidemiologic studies. In fact, the published research shows the opposite. A critical review published in the *Journal of the American College of Nutrition* actually concluded that low-protein diets have adverse effects on bone, whereas higher protein intakes have a *positive* impact. It turns out that the increased calcium in the urine—with higher protein intake—is due to increased absorption of calcium from the intestines. So protein causes more of the calcium you eat to be absorbed, resulting in more calcium available for your bones. Some of this additional calcium may not be needed by your bones, though, and so it's simply excreted, accounting for the mysterious increase in urine calcium on a higher protein diet. It's important to remember, though, that low-carb diets such as TNT are actually high-fat diets, not high-protein.

As far as low-carbohydrate diets specifically, though, a 2006 study conducted at South Florida University determined that a strict low-carb diet—40 grams or less a day—had absolutely no effect on the markers of bone loss or bone formation over a 3-month period. In fact, the low-carb dieters didn't differ in either of these measurements from study participants who consumed a typical American diet.

followed a low-carb diet experienced a 50 percent greater reduction in belly fat than those who ate a low-fat diet. More impressive, though, were the effects seen on the study participants' underlying health.

Because everyone is different, we can't guarantee your results will be as dramatic as those of our participants. But we know that our own lab work as well as the available science shows that by adopting a low-carb diet like TNT, you can quickly battle many of the health problems that are slowly killing millions of Americans every year.

WHAT TO EXPECT

The right diet should, of course, improve your health. And we believe that will happen for most people when they adhere to the guidelines of TNT. There's no doubt that individual results vary, so not everyone will experience the same degree of blood work improvements. But following the TNT Diet, on average, you should anticipate that you will . . .

REDUCE TRIGLYCERIDES BY 51 PERCENT

This is the most consistent response to a low-carb diet. Triglycerides are the chemical name for the form most fat takes in your body. In recent years, the level of blood triglycerides has been shown to be an increasingly important independent risk factor for heart disease. For instance, in a 40-year study, University of Hawaii researchers found that middle-aged men with the lowest triglycerides were the most likely to have "exceptional survival rates." This was defined as living until 85 years of age without suffering from any of six major diseases: coronary heart disease, stroke, cancer, chronic obstructive pulmonary disease, Parkinson's disease, and diabetes.

Of course, you might think that consuming a high amount of fats would boost the amount of fat circulating in your blood. But it turns out that the opposite is true. Remarkably, carbohydrates are more likely to be responsible for dangerously high levels of triglycerides in your bloodstream. Remember how your body converts excess blood sugar to fat in your liver? That fat is triglycerides, which are then transported back into your bloodstream. So by limiting carbohydrates, except for when your glycogen levels are low, you'll automatically lower your triglycerides. In fact, the reduction in blood levels of triglycerides on a low-carb diet are even greater than triglyceride-lowering drugs can achieve.

INCREASE GOOD CHOLESTEROL BY 13 PERCENT

Cholesterol is a well-known factor in cardiovascular disease risk. You're probably familiar with three measurements: LDL, or "bad" cholesterol; HDL, or "good" cholesterol; and total cholesterol, which is roughly the total amount of bad and good cholesterol combined. Most doctors will tell you that it's best to keep your bad cholesterol low and your good cholesterol high. Here's why: LDL cholesterol is believed to lay down plaque in your arteries, while HDL removes plaque.

However, for years, the emphasis in the health-care community has been primarily on lowering both total and LDL cholesterol levels. Why? Because except for exercise, physicians couldn't figure out how to raise the good HDL. So the idea was to treat the risk factors that you *can* improve. And it turns out, in addition to losing weight and taking drugs such as statins, you can decrease total and LDL cholesterol by eating a low-fat diet. Seems like a sensible solution, right? Wrong.

The reason: Along with lowering total and LDL cholesterol, low-fat diets also decrease HDL cholesterol and tend to increase triglycerides (since they're high in carbs). Which brings us back to low-carb diets. As we noted in a recent study, the low-carb approach increases HDL cholesterol by 13 percent and almost always significantly reduces triglycerides. Of course, that leads to the question, What happens to the bad LDL? The answer to that is variable: some people see increases, some observe decreases, and some experience no change. But regardless, because HDL increases significantly more than LDL, your risk of heart disease goes down.

A 2006 study, published in the *American Journal of Cardiology*, reported that your levels of LDL cholesterol only matter in relation to your levels of HDL. For example, let's say your LDL is 100 and your HDL is 30 compared to another guy whose LDL is 150 and HDL is 80. Which one of you has the lowest risk for heart disease? The answer is that it's the other guy, since his ratio of LDL to HDL is far smaller, or better. (To do the calculation yourself, just divide LDL by HDL.) The same math applies to the ratio of total cholesterol to HDL—the lower the number, the lower your risk. It's important to note that this data was derived from the famous Framingham Study. Started in 1948, the Framingham Study is still going strong and is credited with providing most of the knowledge we have today about heart disease risk.

All that said, physicians have been trained to raise their eyebrows in concern when LDL rises even just a little—regardless of any positive change in

HDL. It's important in understanding the TNT Diet that we delve a little deeper into the complexity of cholesterol. And that means understanding that not all LDL cholesterol is created equal. Case in point: LDL particle size, which we'll cover next.

DECREASE THE DEADLIEST CHOLESTEROL BY 10 PERCENT

Contrary to popular opinion, not all LDL cholesterol is bad. Doctors have known for many years that LDL comes in different sizes. There's pattern A, which are large, "fluffy" particles, and pattern B, which are small, dense particles. Back in 1997, Canadian researchers reported for the first time that men with the greatest number of small, dense particles had a nearly four times greater risk for developing heart disease than those with the least number. As they followed these men over the next several years, they confirmed this finding. They also determined that large, fluffy particles of LDL were not even associated with heart disease. So it's not just how much LDL cholesterol you have, it's the type of LDL cholesterol that matters. Bottom line: Small LDL particles have been shown over and over to be associated with increased cardiovascular disease.

Can you guess the number one factor determining LDL size? It turns out it's the carbohydrate content of your diet. You know how enthusiastic we are about low-carbohydrate diets, so you won't be surprised to find out that they change the LDL particles from small to large—that is, from harmful to harmless. Even though total LDL cholesterol may stay the same or even increase slightly with the TNT Diet, the size of those LDL particles increases. As a result, the amount of the small, dense, artery-clogging particles floating around in your bloodstream is reduced, which significantly decreases your risk of heart disease. For example, the low-carb dieters in our lab experienced a 10 percent reduction in small LDL particles. Thus, even if you are one of the people who experiences an increase in LDL cholesterol levels, this is likely due to an increase in the nonthreatening large, fluffy LDL particles. At the same time, you probably also increased HDL cholesterol and reduced your triglycerides—a finding you should share with your doctors should they ever raise their eyebrows at your LDL numbers.

CUT A KEY PREDICTOR OF HEART ATTACKS BY 54 PERCENT

The trouble with asking your doctor to check your LDL particle size is that few will accommodate you—at least not if you're paying with insurance. That's because insurance companies are behind the times when it comes to covering charges for some of the emerging risk factors. But you can probably figure it out for yourself, by calculating your ratio of triglycerides to HDL. To do so, simply divide your triglycerides by your HDL cholesterol reading. Researchers at the Albert Einstein College of Medicine determined that this ratio is inversely related to LDL particle size. That means the lower your ratio, the larger and fluffier your LDL particles. For instance, scientists found that 83 percent of people whose ratio was 3.8 or greater had a predominance of small, dense LDL particles, compared with just 11 percent of those whose ratio was lower. Let's walk through an example. Suppose your triglycerides are 125, and your HDL cholesterol is 50. You'd divide 125 by 50, for a triglyceride-HDL ratio of 2.5. Congratulations: Your LDL particles are as big and fluffy as the Stay-Puft Marshmallow Man.

In addition, the triglyceride-HDL ratio is also strongly correlated with insulin resistance, according to Stanford University researchers. The scientists found that people with the highest ratio have eight times the risk for a heart attack than those with the lowest. Thankfully, we've found that low-carb diets lower this ratio by an average of 54 percent.

LOWER YOUR BLOOD SUGAR BY 12 PERCENT

A person has normal blood sugar when his fasting glucose—the most common gauge—is between 70 and 100 milligrams per deciliter (mg/dl). He's considered diabetic when that number reaches 126 mg/dl. In between the two is what's known as *impaired fasting glucose,* or prediabetes. Prediabetes is such an accurate predictor of future diabetes that 95 percent of people in this category end up with the disease.

High blood sugar, also called *hyperglycemia,* has been shown to damage both the small blood vessels of your eyes and kidneys—which is why diabetes is linked to blindness and renal failure—as well as the larger vessels that deliver blood to your heart. The latter helps explain the connection between diabetes and heart disease. In fact, Johns Hopkins researchers determined that high blood sugar is now an independent risk for heart disease. It's also an indicator of insulin resistance. But here's the good news: In a recent study, we found that a low-carb diet, like TNT, lowers blood sugar by 12 percent in 12 weeks. This is a huge health benefit to someone who has high blood sugar. That's because it can help a guy with prediabetes quickly restore his blood sugar to normal levels, which instantly reduces his risk of heart disease, diabetes, and kidney disease.

SLASH INSULIN BY 48 PERCENT

When you consider that insulin resistance results in high insulin levels, it's not hard to understand why lower insulin levels are an indicator of improved health. Don't misunderstand: Insulin isn't bad—it's necessary for life. And as we've shown, it can be used at certain times to effectively build muscle. The trouble comes when insulin is chronically elevated. Doctors determine this by measuring insulin after you've fasted for at least 8 hours. Since you've had no food—such as carbohydrates—insulin shouldn't be elevated. When it is, this is a sign of insulin resistance, as well as future heart disease and diabetes. Of course, chronically elevated insulin levels also keep your body in a perpetual fat-storing mode, leading to larger visceral fat cells, which can cause even more health problems. However, low-carb diets are extremely effective at reducing fasting insulin levels—cutting them almost in half.

LOWER INFLAMMATION BY 55 PERCENT

Over the last few years, it's been determined that inflammation may be one of the best indicators of future heart disease and many other afflictions, such as cancer. One of the most recognized and well-studied markers of inflammation is a blood compound known as *C-reactive protein* (CRP). In fact, scientists now believe that elevated levels of CRP are highly predictive of looming heart disease. That's why we measured it in a recent low-carb study at our lab. The result: Men eating a low-carb diet experienced a 55 percent reduction in CRP. In addition, we measured several other markers of inflammation, all of which decreased when people cut back on carbs. Clearly, low-carb diets such as TNT are naturally anti-inflammatory. Which means they offer protection from many diseases.

MUSCLE CAN SAVE YOUR LIFE

Indulge us for a moment and flex your right arm. Assuming you have an average build, you're looking at about 6 pounds of muscle. That hard figure might sound disappointing, but it's hardly minuscule; it represents about 10 percent of the total muscle on your body.

Now imagine that muscle gone. No biceps, no triceps, no wrist flexors—only a jiggly mass of skin and fat covering your bones from your shoulder down to your fingertips. Simply put, you'd be a mess. But consider this: As we noted earlier, that 6 pounds of muscle is the same amount most men lose between the ages of 30 and 50. And that number doubles by time they're 60.

In fact, once a man passes the half-century mark, he can expect to lose 1 percent of his muscle each year for the rest of his life.

Carrying around extra fat only makes this worse. Researchers at the National Institutes of Health found that some of the adipokines that fat cells secrete signal your body to break down muscle tissue. Specifically, interleukin-6, an inflammatory agent that's been linked to a decline in strength and mobility, particularly in people with high amounts of visceral fat. Although the scientists aren't sure why interleukin-6 may cause muscle loss, they speculate that it could be because it inhibits muscle-building hormones. It's also thought that high levels of interleukin-6 may cause insulin resistance, which means your muscles won't respond to the effects of insulin. That's critical, you'll remember, because insulin helps to ensure your muscles aren't broken down and used for energy.

If all of this doesn't scare the hell out of you, it should. Life without muscle is miserable and short. That's because the natural erosion of muscle as you age, and the loss of strength that accompanies it, lead directly to weak bones, stiff joints, and poor posture. Muscle loss also increases your risk for heart disease and diabetes, and makes it less likely that you'll recover from a serious

Do You Have Metabolic Syndrome?

To know whether or not you suffer from metabolic syndrome, you'll need to have a blood test done by your family doctor. If you meet at least three out of the five criteria listed below, then you meet the definition of metabolic syndrome. That said, if any of these markers are not in the normal range, you should monitor them closely throughout the TNT program. We recommend having your blood retested every 8 to 12 weeks.

RISK FACTOR	DEFINING LEVEL
Abdominal Obesity (waist circumference)	
Men	>40 in
Women	>35 in
HDL Cholesterol	
Men	<40 mg/dl
Women	<50 mg/dl
Triglycerides	≥150 mg/dl
Glucose	≥100 mg/dl
Blood Pressure	
Systolic (top number)	≥130 mmHg
Diastolic (bottom number)	≥85 mmHg

disease, such as cancer. Your once-strong, healthy body is transformed into that of a frail—and soon to be dead—old man.

But you don't have to accept that fate. Instead of helplessly letting your muscle—and your life—waste away, you can defend both from the ravages of time with help from the best anti-aging weapon in any man's arsenal: resistance training. Regularly lifting weights signals your body to fight for your muscle. That means a longer, healthier life. And besides making you fit and strong, the actual process of training your muscles with weights provides many benefits. This is one of the many reasons we've made weight training a key component in the TNT plan. Without it, you'd be shortchanging your body, and shortchanging your health. In fact, doing three total-body work-outs a week—like the ones found in Chapter 11—will help you:

Keep your heart healthy. Researchers at the University of Michigan found that men who performed three total-body weight workouts per week for 2 months lowered their diastolic blood pressure (the bottom number) by an average of eight points. That's enough to reduce the risk of a stroke by 40 percent, and the risk of a heart attack by 15 percent.

Build stronger bones. Just like muscle, you lose bone mass as you age, too, increasing the likelihood you'll one day suffer a debilitating fracture in your hips or vertebrae. That's even worse than it sounds, since Mayo Clinic researchers found that 30 percent of men die within 1 year of breaking a hip. In addition, significant bone loss in your spine can result in perpetually rounded shoulders and the dreaded "dowager's hump," a condi-tion that literally transforms you into a 21st-century Quasimodo. The good news: A study in the *Journal of Applied Physiology* found that 16 weeks of resis-tance training increased hip bone density in men, and elevated blood levels of osteocalcin—a marker of bone growth—by 19 percent.

Increase your flexibility. Between the ages of 30 and 70, flexibility decreases 20 to 50 percent. That results in an inability for you to move through a joint's full range of motion. For example, if you can't squat down until the back of your thighs touch your calves (most men can't), you have tight hip flexors, which limits your movement at the knee joint. In a study published in the *International Journal of Sports Medicine,* researchers found that three full-body workouts a week for 16 weeks increased flexibility of the hips and shoulders by more than 30 percent, while improving sit-and-reach test scores by 11 percent. Not convinced that weight training doesn't leave you "muscle-bound"? Research shows that Olympic weight lifters rate only second to gymnasts in overall flexibility.

Reduce diabetes risk. Every time you eat sugary foods or processed carbohydrates such as white bread, rice, and potatoes, your levels of insulin rise dramatically. That's a problem because consistently elevated insulin increases your risk for diabetes and heart disease. But weights can help: Researchers at the University of Massachusetts found that men who added two full-body weight workouts a week to their existing aerobic exercise program had 25 percent lower insulin levels after a sugary meal than men who performed the same aerobic exercise program, but didn't lift weights.

Stay in the game. It's not just the quantity of the muscle you lose that's important, it's the quality. Research shows that your fast-twitch muscle fibers are reduced by up to 50 percent as you age, while slow-twitch fibers decrease less than 25 percent. It's important because fast-twitch fibers are the muscles largely responsible for generating strength and power. These muscles hold the key to peak sports performance when you're young and help you easily get out of a chair when you're old. Another benefit: Researchers in Georgia found that men with osteoarthritis who performed leg exercises through a full range of motion three times a week reduced knee pain by up to 58 percent.

Fight cancer. High levels of visceral fat increase your risk for both prostate and colon cancer. However, researchers in Spain found that men who simply participated in a twice-weekly weight-training program for 4 months decreased visceral fat stores by 10 percent, reducing disease risk. And in a study published in *Medicine and Science in Sports and Exercise,* scientists found that resistance training speeds the rate at which food is moved through your large intestine by up to 56 percent, an effect that's thought to reduce the risk for colon cancer.

Waists and Measures

Tracking your waist circumference is an easy way to gauge your progress—and your risk for heart disease. Here's how to do it: Wrap a measuring tape around your abdomen—or better yet, have someone help you—so that the bottom of the tape touches the tops of your hip bones. (Your belly button moves as you lose fat, but your hip bones don't; so this method ensures that you always take the measurement at the exact same location.) The tape should be snug, but shouldn't compress the skin, and should be parallel to the floor. If the tape measures 36 inches or greater, you need to take action. Today.

Lead a happier life. In a 2004 study at the University of Alabama-Birmingham, researchers found that older men who performed three weight workouts a week for 6 months improved their scores on measures of confusion, tension, anger, and overall mood. Although unsure of the mechanism, study author Gary Hunter, PhD, suggests, "It could simply be a feeling of accomplishment from having become fit and more confident in themselves." Makes sense: The study participants reversed a decade of age-related muscle loss and fat gain, by adding 4 pounds of muscle and dropping 3 pounds of fat, while increasing strength by an average of 42 percent. Those results would improve anyone's mood.

CHAPTER 13

SATURATED FAT AND THE AMERICAN PARADOX

Paradox (păr'ə-dŏks') *n.* A statement that seems contradictory or absurd but is actually valid or true.

Imagine this headline: Eating More Saturated Fat Lowers the Risk for Heart Disease.

Inconceivable? For most people, the answer would be yes. The headline contradicts the widely held belief that saturated fat is a direct cause of heart disease and diabetes—that it is, in fact, a dietary demon. Yet this very headline described the recent findings of a Harvard University study. The scientists reported that people who had the highest saturated fat intake also had the *least* plaque buildup on their artery walls. As a result, heart disease risk was lowest in those who consumed the most saturated fat. These results were so counterintuitive that a scientific editorial published in the *American Journal of Clinical Nutrition* described the findings as an "American paradox."

On the surface, the positive results of increased saturated fat may seem puzzling, but it's not without precedence. After all, the "French paradox" was discovered in 1981, when researchers noted that the people of France had very low death rates from coronary heart disease, despite consuming high amounts of saturated fat. (Just think foie gras and brie.) Could these findings have simply been scientific anomalies? Or is it that conventional wisdom about saturated fat is based on a false set of assumptions? A closer look at this misunderstood nutrient reveals a new paradigm—one that provides a clear explanation for the paradox that most people believe is a contradiction.

THE WRONG PARADIGM

Did you know there are over a dozen different types of saturated fat in the human diet? Not many people do. Turns out, different types of saturated fat have varying effects on your cholesterol levels. For instance, some saturated fats actually have no impact on cholesterol. And while other types may raise LDL (bad) cholesterol, almost all saturated fats simultaneously boost HDL (good) cholesterol to an even greater extent, resulting in a lower risk of heart disease.

Typically, though, saturated fats are lumped into a single category: Unhealthy. In fact, for most health-conscious Americans, the mere mention of saturated fat conjures up images of waxy streaks in meat and narrowing arteries in our chests. That's the message that has been commonly put forth by the nation's top health organizations for more than 40 years. Because of this message, saturated fat has effectively been branded the main culprit for nearly every diet-related disease, including obesity, diabetes, heart disease, and cancer. But considering how aggressively the evils of saturated fat have been sold to the American public, it's worth exploring the evidence that supports these assertions.

The message to reduce saturated fat originated decades ago, based mainly on observations made by a well-known scientist named Ancel Keys. In 1953, Keys published a paper that showed an association between fat intake and coronary heart disease deaths across populations living in six different countries. For instance, Japan had the lowest fat intakes, and the fewest number of deaths from heart disease. The United States, on the other hand, had the highest fat intake, and the most deaths from heart disease. In 1958, Keys published another study, this time suggesting that fat intake was linked to blood cholesterol levels in various societies. The more fat people ate, the higher their cholesterol. And a few years later, he reported that this correlation was even stronger when one compared animal fat intake—the main source of saturated fat in our diets—as opposed to total fat intake. All of this led to the "diet-heart hypothesis," which proposed that the higher a person's saturated fat intake, the higher the risk for heart disease.

Given Keys's findings and the scientific knowledge at the time, the diet-heart hypothesis seemed to make sense. After all, dietary saturated fat was known to elevate total cholesterol levels (A), and elevated total cholesterol levels (B) were associated with increased heart disease (C). In other words, if A caused B, and B caused C, then A must logically cause C. Or so one might think. But this type of logic can often lead to false conclusions. Consider this example: Exercise causes increased blood pressure. Elevated blood pressure increases risk of heart disease. Therefore, exercise causes heart disease. Obviously this is a ridiculous conclusion, but the same logic was used to condemn saturated fat.

Of course, this doesn't mean that Keys was necessarily wrong. But a closer look at the science behind this hypothesis yields some startling revelations. For example, Keys's original 1953 study looked at data from only six countries. Yet at the time, statistics were available for 22 countries. This was pointed out in a 1957 paper by two scientists, Jacob Yerushalmy, PhD, and Herman Hilleboe, MD, who analyzed the data from all 22 countries—Keys's original 6, plus the 16 that were somehow overlooked. The result: Dr. Yerushalmy and Dr. Hilleboe determined that there was no longer a clear connection between fat intake and deaths from coronary heart disease. The countries that Keys didn't include significantly weakened the association between the pats of butter that Americans were eating and the clogged arteries that were killing us. In fact, additional research found that consumption of sugar was more strongly correlated with heart disease than animal fat. In addition, cigarette smoking, owning a car, and animal protein consumption were all more strongly tied to heart disease than total fat intake.

Could it be that Keys's other studies were similarly flawed, perhaps even biased? Consider his most well-known work, the Seven Countries Study, which was published in 1970. In the study, Keys selected seven countries and determined that animal fat intake was the best predictor of heart attacks over a 5-year period. For example, Finnish men had five times greater incidence of heart disease than the Japanese, which Keys attributed to their diets—men living in Finland ate significantly more animal fat than those living in Japan.

But consider this: During the study, there were five times more fatal heart attacks and twice the rate of heart disease in western Finland compared to eastern Finland, despite only small differences in animal fat intake. Although Keys addresses this finding in his paper, it amounts to little more than a footnote, in which he suggests that future research will provide the explanation for this disconnect. However, as Danish scientist Uffe Ravnskov, MD, PhD, points out in his book, *The Cholesterol Myths,* this illustrates a continuing problem with the "science" that has led to the idea that eating saturated fat causes heart disease. "Observations that support the theory are trumpeted as positive proofs while unsupportive findings, if they are mentioned at all, are considered 'rare exceptions' or 'something that cannot be explained,'" Dr. Ravnskov writes.

For example, had Ancel Keys studied other countries, such as France, or individual societies, like the Masai tribe in Kenya, the Inuit of Northern Canada and Greenland, and the Fulani of Nigeria, he would have drawn very different conclusions. Each of these cultures ate high amounts of fat and saturated fat, and yet cardiovascular disease was virtually nonexistent.

Take the Fulani, a tribe of seminomadic pastoralists in northern Nigeria. In a 2001 study, University of New Mexico researchers found that although the Fulani consumed nearly 50 percent of their calories from fat—half of which was saturated—cholesterol levels were "normal," and they had a very low incidence of heart disease. It's important to point out that the Fulani were also lean, very physically active, and didn't overeat. They also had low rates of smoking and alcohol consumption.

Which makes one wonder, is it really the saturated fat that causes heart disease, or other factors, such as overall lifestyle, including the basic fact that we eat too much and exercise too little? Today, no one will argue that as diets and lifestyles around the world have become "Westernized," the prevalence of heart disease has risen. This Westernization includes higher rates of smoking and obesity, as well as a greater intake of processed foods, particularly carbohydrates.

You can even see the effect in the United States: Since the 1970s, saturated fat intake has decreased by 14 percent in men, while carbohydrate consumption has increased by 23 percent. Yet rates of heart disease, along with obesity, are skyrocketing. If we were to simply make an assumption based on observational data, like Keys, we might conclude that carbohydrates make people fat, which leads to heart disease. Or we might just say that the more carbohydrates you eat, the greater your risk for a heart attack.

However, as we've pointed out with Keys's data, there are too many factors to make sweeping generalizations. That is, unless you also can provide physiological evidence that supports your assertion.

Population studies, as we've shown, only *suggest* causal relationships. To prove them, you need to be able to replicate the findings in a controlled experiment. For example, you could analyze a group of people's dietary intake to determine how much saturated fat they were eating, and then measure their blood for heart disease risk factors.

Once you've gathered their baseline data, you could then have half of the people decrease their saturated fat intake, while the others make no changes to their diet.

Monitor these people for a certain period of time, and you could then see the effect of this one dietary change on not only risk factors, but on the development of heart disease itself. This, although not without its flaws, is a far more accurate way to determine risk than a population study. And it turns out, this kind of study has been done—many times. The only problem: None of these clinical trials has shown that decreasing saturated fat intake reduces heart disease risk. Nor is there a clear, decisive study that has ever demonstrated the diet-heart hypothesis to be true. Not that scientists haven't tried. Over the last five decades, research costing billions of dollars has been conducted in an effort to prove that saturated fat causes heart disease. And yet every single study has turned up empty. If the diet-heart hypothesis were true, don't you think there would be a smoking gun? People promoting low-fat diets thought for sure that they would have one in the Women's Health Initiative.

The Women's Health Initiative (WHI) is by far the largest clinical trial funded by our federal government. The WHI was designed to show once and for all the clear benefits of limiting both total and saturated fat intake on heart disease and even cancer risk. In the study, nearly 50,000 postmenopausal women were divided into two groups: One group focused on decreasing total dietary fat and saturated fat, the other group made no dietary changes. Over an average of 6 years, the low-fat dieters ate 29 percent less saturated fat than those who didn't change their eating habits. The findings: Reducing saturated fat didn't decrease the incidence of heart disease, stroke, or cancer. In fact, the percentage of both nonfatal heart attacks and deaths from coronary heart disease were exactly the same in both groups.

Now, you might think this would spur a critical rethinking of the original diet-heart hypothesis. But instead, the lead researchers on the project took the peculiar position that the women failed to restrict saturated fat enough to improve health. As such, the ensuing newspaper headlines reflected this dubious conclusion, and most health professionals adopted this viewpoint. Keep in mind, though, that the 29 percent difference in saturated fat intake between the groups of women was calculated to meet the highest standards of statistical significance. Which means the scientific conclusion was that significantly decreasing saturated fat intake had no impact on heart disease.

SATURATED FAT: THE BENEFITS TO YOUR BODY

Where then does the misguided diet-heart hypothesis go wrong? There are two major problems that are rarely considered. First, saturated fat does much more than just impact total cholesterol levels. In fact, many of these other effects actually improve overall health. And you get these benefits even if you don't lose weight or exercise.

Second, the impact of saturated fat has to be considered along with carbohydrate intake. Remember our examples of the Inuit and Fulani? They eat lots of saturated fat, but very few carbs. They also have a low incidence of heart disease. So when examining the effect of saturated fat on health, it's imperative to also look at the intake of carbohydrates as well.

Here are some of the facts about saturated fat that are not so well known. You'll notice that many of the facts also relate to eating a low-carb diet.

• Replacing carbohydrates with saturated fat—or any type of fat—results in decreased triglycerides levels, an independent risk factor for heart disease. We've shown this time and time again in our published studies.

• Replacing carbohydrates with saturated fat—or again, any type of fat—results in increased HDL (good) cholesterol levels. In fact, saturated fat raises HDL even more than unsaturated fat.

• Saturated fat increases the size of LDL particles, which are a less atherogenic, or harmful, form of LDL cholesterol.

• Not all saturated fats raise cholesterol. For instance, stearic acid—a type of saturated fatty acid found in meats—has a neutral effect on LDL cholesterol. (See "The Truth about Steak" on page 238.)

These facts, which often run contrary to what you've been led to believe, have been proven through well-controlled studies conducted over the last decade in our lab and many others. They hold far more weight than observational findings from population studies. Yet for some reason, many scientists and health professionals dismiss them because they contradict the decades-old diet-heart hypothesis—a proposition that is based on questionable data and has never been proven.

A NEW PARADIGM

Are you ready for the "mother" of all outrageous paradoxes? Eating more saturated fat actually results in decreased blood levels of saturated fat. That's not a typographical error. We recently conducted a tightly controlled diet study where we had overweight men and women follow either a low-carb or low-fat diet for 12 weeks. Before and after our experiment, we performed

day, rate the following, on a scale of 1 (most favorable) to 7 (least favorable):

- Your ability to work without stopping to take unscheduled breaks.

- Your ability to stick to your routine or plan (your to-do list) for the day.

- Your overall job performance.

"It's likely you'll find that you score higher and get more done on the days you exercise, despite taking time out for your workout," says Dr. McKenna. And that means you'll have greater motivation to stick with it.

This is just one basic example. But see how it all works? You can use a similar template for virtually every aspect of your life, including the TNT Diet. All you have to do is create a checklist of items that you want to track. The obvious one that most people choose is weight. But suppose you monitor your mood, energy level, general wellness (Did you catch a cold? How long did it last?), and work productivity. And don't forget chronic problems that you already have—it could be the aforementioned regular headaches, heartburn, acne, canker sores (all of which low-carb diets help relieve), or even anxiety. Make sure to note if there is an onset of any of these after you start your plan as well. We've provided a sample journal on page 246.

Also, it's imperative you give your body some time to adapt. So you'll need to stick with your program for a decent period of time—let's say 4 to 6 weeks—before coming to any conclusions. (And, of course, you've hopefully already decided to stay with it for the full 12 weeks.) This will give you a sufficient period to gather information. It's also helpful to have baseline data, so you may want to track yourself for a week or two before you actually start your plan.

Relieve Heartburn

University of North Carolina scientists reported that within 4 days of initiating a low-carbohydrate diet, overweight patients experienced a 53 percent reduction in the severity of heartburn-like symptoms. What's more, the pain-causing acid in each person's esophagus decreased by an average of 39 percent. The scientists aren't sure why reducing carbohydrates worked, but report that in a previous study, patients' symptoms returned once they returned to a carbohydrate-heavy diet.

WEEK 1	MON	TUES	WED	THURS	FRI	SAT	SUN
Other (any other ailments that you regularly experience, or any that commence— note them below)							
Sleep (quality, on scale of 1 to 10, 1 being the best night's sleep, 10 being the worst)							
Mood (quality, on scale of 1 to 10, 1 being the best mood, 10 being the worst)							
Work productivity (from 1 to 7, 1 being the best, 7 being the worst)							
Ability to work without stopping to take unscheduled breaks							
Ability to stick to your routine or plan (your to-do list) for the day							
Overall job performance							

Dietary intake is straightforward: You control it by how much fat you put in your mouth. However, the production of new saturated fat is a bit more complicated. This manufacturing process is triggered by the hormone insulin. As you recall from earlier chapters, insulin levels rise when you eat carbohydrates, and this signals your body to stop burning—and start storing—fat. But there's one thing you don't know yet: Insulin also tells your body to increase the production of fat in your liver. And it turns out, the main type of fat made in your liver is indeed the saturated kind. That means that the more carbs you eat, the more saturated fat your body makes.

So what happens when you eat a low-carbohydrate diet? Your insulin levels are lower and the production of saturated fatty acids is dramatically reduced, of course.

There's another benefit to low-carb diets. Since they keep insulin levels low, they allow your body to burn more fat—including saturated fat—for energy. This decreases your body's saturated fat pool even further.

Viewed in this context, the apparent paradox, "a higher saturated fat intake decreases blood levels of saturated fat," actually makes perfect sense. When your carbohydrate intake is low, your body makes less saturated fat, and is better able to burn the saturated fat that you consume. The end result is a remarkable reduction in the amount of saturated fat circulating in your bloodstream.

The take-home message: Saturated fat is not the villain to your health that everyone is making it out to be.

CHAPTER 14

TNT FOR LIFE

aking your shirt off in public is purely optional—and generally frowned upon. So if your diet and exercise plan's only purpose is to help you finally achieve six-pack abs (or even just a two-pack), it may be hard to stick with for the long haul.

But while we aren't behaviorists, we've recently observed a process that we think can help anyone institute lasting lifestyle changes—particularly when it comes to fitness and nutrition. The key, we believe, is to provide yourself with additional motivators, such as your health and overall well-being. But you have to think beyond cholesterol. For instance, you should start by monitoring recurring health issues that you already have—like migraines, heartburn, acne, canker sores, and poor sleep quality—along with blood pressure, cholesterol, triglycerides, and other common measures of cardiovascular health. After all, discovering that your diet or exercise regimen helps relieve the symptoms of a longtime ailment, and improves the quality of your everyday life, can be a powerful source of motivation.

Let's say you have recurring migraines, a frustrating and painful problem that's plagued you for several years. Now imagine if you discovered that avoiding certain foods completely eliminated this ailment. Would you do it? Chances are, you would—and probably without a second thought. You see, once you're given the proper motivation to stick to a specific diet, it becomes very easy to follow. We speak from personal experience because both of us have had these types of breakthrough experiences. We've also seen the same impact on the lives of many other men and women.

It's important to note that the hard part about a low-carb diet, like the one you'll follow in the Fat-Burning Time Zone, is simply the knowledge that there are great-tasting foods out there—for instance, sugar—that you can't eat. But if you can determine that the quality of your life improves dramatically without them, then those tasty foods become inconsequential compared

(continued on page 244)

Conquer Your Cravings

Because we can all use as much good advice as possible, we asked a few of our friends and colleagues for their best tips on how to stick with your eating plan. They didn't disappoint us.

Guarantee Success

Before you initiate your diet, perform a reality check: How long do you *honestly* think you can stick to it? Start with 4 weeks, and work your way down—for instance, 3 weeks, 2 weeks, 3 days—until you've found a duration that you're 100 percent confident you can achieve, even if it's just a couple of days. "Once you make it to your goal-date, start the process over," says Mary Vernon, MD, president of the American Society of Bariatric Physicians. "This not only establishes that you can be successful, but it also gives you a chance to start noticing that eating better makes you feel better, reinforcing your desire to continue."

Don't Dwell on Mistakes

See if this sounds familiar: You've successfully followed your diet for a few days, but then you hit a glitch—in the form of, say, the entire wall menu at Taco Bell. What's the next step? "Forget about it," says James Newman, a nutritionist at Tahlequah City Hospital in Oklahoma, who used his own advice to shed 275 pounds. (That's right: 275 pounds.) "One meal doesn't define your diet, so don't assume that you've failed or fallen off the wagon," he says. After all, in how many other areas of your life do you achieve perfection? To make sure a one-time slipup doesn't snowball into a face-feeding free-for-all, institute a simple rule: Pledge to follow any "cheat" meal with at least five meals and snacks that meet your criteria for a healthy diet. That ensures that you'll be eating right more than 80 percent of the time.

Eat Breakfast

Sure, you've heard this one before. But it's important: Researchers at the University of Massachusetts found that men who don't eat breakfast are nearly five times more likely to be obese than those who make it an everyday habit. And timing matters: Make sure you eat your first meal within 1 hour and 18 minutes of waking. The scientists determined that guys who waited a half-hour longer increased the likelihood that they'd become heavyweights by 147 percent; those that didn't eat breakfast within 3 hours of waking elevated their risk by 173 percent.

Why is holding off on your first meal so bad? Consider that if you sleep for 6 to 8 hours, and then skip breakfast, your body is essentially running on fumes by the time you get to work. And that sends you desperately seeking sugar, which happens to be easy to find. Which brings us to our next strategy . . .

Install Food Regulators

The only things worse than a pantry and refrigerator full of blood-sugar-raising junk food are those that are empty. So clean out your cupboard and fridge, then re-stock them with almonds (and other nuts), cheese, fruit, vegetables, and canned tuna and chicken. And do the same at work. "By eliminating snacks that don't match your diet, but providing plenty that do, you're far less likely to find yourself at the doughnut shop drive-thru or the vending machine," says Christopher Mohr, PhD, RD, owner of Mohr Results in Louisville, Kentucky. One other trick: Pre-portion servings of snack foods such as nuts into plastic bags, as opposed to eating them out of the jar.

Think Like a Biochemist

It's true: They make all-natural cookies. But even if a cookie is made with organic cane juice (aka a hippie name for sugar), it's still junk food. That's because just like the "bad" stuff, it raises your blood sugar. "If you're going to eat a cookie, accept that you're deviating from your plan, and then revert to your diet afterward," says Valerie Berkowitz, MS, RD, director of nutrition at the Center for Balanced Health in New York City. "By convincing yourself that it's healthy, you're only encouraging a bad habit." Of course, if you're in the Reloading Time Zone, you can get away with a cookie here and there, without doing damage. Our advice: Eat the kind you like, even if it's not made with hippie sugar.

Recognize Hunger

Have a craving for sweets, even though you just ate an hour ago? Imagine eating a large sizzling steak instead. "If you're truly hungry, the steak will sound good, and you should eat," says Richard Feinman, PhD, professor of biochemistry at SUNY Downstate Medical Center in New York City. "If it doesn't sound good, your brain is playing tricks on you."

His advice: Have a hard-cooked egg or a slice of cheese, and then wait a few minutes. Still not working? Then it's time to change your environment, which can be as easy as doing 15 pushups (close your office door), or finding a different task to focus on. One caveat: "Avoid activities, such as paying your bills, that might make you nervous or uptight, triggering your desire to eat," says Dr. Feinman.

Take a Logical Approach

"Before you take a bite of food, consider whether it's taking you one step closer to your goals or one step further away," says Alwyn Cosgrove, MS, CSCS. This won't stop you from making a poor choice every single time, but it does encourage the habit of thinking about what you eat. The payoff: "Eighty to 90 percent of the time you'll make a better decision."

to all the other benefits you experience by avoiding them. Think of it like this: At some point, usually in college, many of us find out the hard way that drinking too much tequila can have pretty negative consequences, unless, that is, you enjoy resting your head on porcelain. You could call it a conditioned response: Get sick on tequila once and you quickly develop a natural repulsion to it. Maybe it's the same way with diet and exercise. When you realize that a food is making you feel bad, you're more likely to avoid it. Or, when you realize how good a low-carbohydrate diet and regular exercise can make you feel, you're more likely to embrace it.

Now here's our premise: Everyone that's able to stick with a specific type of diet or exercise program permanently probably has had a moment of revelation—that time when he realizes that the benefits of the lifestyle change reach beyond those of vanity. Because, let's face it, at a certain point, the desire for six-pack abs decreases with every passing year. So to make a lasting habit, you need a motivation that's lasting.

Assuming that makes sense, here's the problem: Most of us aren't very good at recognizing the signals our bodies are giving us. Or perhaps more accurately, we aren't very good at matching a positive signal (more energy) or negative signal (a rise in blood pressure) with a specific action we've taken—such as changing our diet.

The solution? You need to develop a process that helps you identify the positive and negative feedback your body is giving you on a daily basis. This will help you to more quickly and accurately figure out the diet and exercise program that works best for your body. And more importantly, it will provide you with hard data with which to fuel your motivation to follow through in the long term.

One of the best examples of this is a study conducted at Leeds Metropolitan University in the United Kingdom, in which the researchers examined how exercise impacts job performance. It worked like this: Each day for a month, 210 workers participating in an exercise program provided daily feedback on job-related duties and time management, as well as on interactions with co-workers. They simply reported observations of their own behavior based on a seven-point scale. For example, they were asked to rate their ability to work without stopping for unscheduled breaks, and how effectively they were able to stick to their "to-do" list for the day. They also provided details about their workload and exercise session. When the results were tallied, even the researchers were surprised.

Consistently, the workers scored 15 percent higher in their ability to meet both time and output demands on the days they exercised compared to when they weren't physically active. They were also 15 percent more tolerant of their co-workers. "What we found staggered us, and we were left wondering what companies might do otherwise to produce these 15 percent improvements," says Jim McKenna, PhD, the lead researcher of the study.

Now consider for a moment what these numbers mean to you: On days you exercise, you can—theoretically at least—accomplish in an 8-hour day what normally would take you 9 hours and 12 minutes. Or you'd still work 9 hours, but get more done, leaving you feeling less stressed and happier with your job, another perk that Dr. McKenna says the workers reported on the days they exercised.

Obviously, the responses that led to all of these results were subjective. But it's hard to deny that perception is reality when it comes to job satisfaction. And a 15 percent boost in productivity might just give you a case for a similar boost in pay.

So let's say that you want to start exercising, but you just can't find the time. This study shows that if you actually take the time to exercise anyway, and then document your work productivity daily, you'll discover that you actually get more done. The end result: Your favorite excuse to not exercise will no longer exist. In fact, you'll now be more motivated to exercise than ever—there's absolutely no downside, and your life should be vastly improved.

For instance, if you want to try this, you'd keep an on-the-job performance journal on both the days you exercise and the days you don't. Each

(continued on page 248)

The Headache Medicine

Cutting back on carbs may relieve you of more than a few extra pounds. In a new study, researchers at Albert Einstein College of Medicine found that low-carb diets help reduce the frequency and severity of headaches in regular sufferers. "Half of those surveyed said they attained the same kind of relief from low-carb diets as they did from a migraine medication," says study author C.J. Segal-Isaacson, EdD, RD. Although the scientists aren't sure why a low-carb prescription helps headaches, they speculate that some people may be more sensitive to carbohydrates and the allergens they contain—such as gluten, a wheat protein. Take note of when your headaches occur: Forty percent of the patients reported pain after eating starchy or sugary foods.

The TNT Wellness Journal

WEEK 1	MON	TUES	WED	THURS	FRI	SAT	SUN
Acne (degree, from 1 to 10, 1 being the least severe, and 10 being the most, or occurrence, along with duration)							
Skin rash (degree, from 1 to 10, 1 being the least severe, and 10 being the most, or occurrence, along with duration)							
Migraines (number each day and severity—on a scale of 1 to 10, 1 being the least severe, 10 being the most)							
Headaches (number each day and severity—on a scale of 1 to 10, 1 being the least severe, 10 being the most)							
Heartburn (number of times each day and severity—on a scale of 1 to 10, 1 being the least severe, 10 being the most)							
Canker sores (when each occurs, and when it has healed by)							
Cold sores (when each occurs, and when it has healed by)							

WEEK 1	MON	TUES	WED	THURS	FRI	SAT	SUN
Other (any other ailments that you regularly experience, or any that commence—note them below)							
Sleep (quality, on scale of 1 to 10, 1 being the best night's sleep, 10 being the worst)							
Mood (quality, on scale of 1 to 10, 1 being the best mood, 10 being the worst)							
Work productivity (from 1 to 7, 1 being the best, 7 being the worst)							
Ability to work without stopping to take unscheduled breaks							
Ability to stick to your routine or plan (your to-do list) for the day							
Overall job performance							

day, rate the following, on a scale of 1 (most favorable) to 7 (least favorable):

- Your ability to work without stopping to take unscheduled breaks.

- Your ability to stick to your routine or plan (your to-do list) for the day.

- Your overall job performance.

"It's likely you'll find that you score higher and get more done on the days you exercise, despite taking time out for your workout," says Dr. McKenna. And that means you'll have greater motivation to stick with it.

This is just one basic example. But see how it all works? You can use a similar template for virtually every aspect of your life, including the TNT Diet. All you have to do is create a checklist of items that you want to track. The obvious one that most people choose is weight. But suppose you monitor your mood, energy level, general wellness (Did you catch a cold? How long did it last?), and work productivity. And don't forget chronic problems that you already have—it could be the aforementioned regular headaches, heartburn, acne, canker sores (all of which low-carb diets help relieve), or even anxiety. Make sure to note if there is an onset of any of these after you start your plan as well. We've provided a sample journal on page 246.

Also, it's imperative you give your body some time to adapt. So you'll need to stick with your program for a decent period of time—let's say 4 to 6 weeks—before coming to any conclusions. (And, of course, you've hopefully already decided to stay with it for the full 12 weeks.) This will give you a sufficient period to gather information. It's also helpful to have baseline data, so you may want to track yourself for a week or two before you actually start your plan.

Relieve Heartburn

University of North Carolina scientists reported that within 4 days of initiating a low-carbohydrate diet, overweight patients experienced a 53 percent reduction in the severity of heartburn-like symptoms. What's more, the pain-causing acid in each person's esophagus decreased by an average of 39 percent. The scientists aren't sure why reducing carbohydrates worked, but report that in a previous study, patients' symptoms returned once they returned to a carbohydrate-heavy diet.

Using this process will better allow you to determine the effect that the TNT Diet is having on your entire life, not just your body. And really, isn't that the whole point? Start listening to your body, and you'll not only learn what you should be doing, but you'll *want* to do it—for the rest of your life.

INDEX

Underscored page references indicate boxed text and tables. **Boldface** references indicate photographs.

A

Abdominal fat
  from carbohydrates, 17, 18
  health effects from, 215
  losing, 12, 221
Acomplia, 217
Adipokines
  in fat, 215
  muscle loss from, 226
Advanced Workout. *See also specific exercises*
  purpose of, 149
  for weeks 1 through 4, 161
  for weeks 5 through 8, 162
  for weeks 9 through 12, 163
Aerobic exercise, 144–45. *See also* Cardio
      workouts
Afterburn effect, 133
Aging, muscle loss with, 3, 225–26
Aioli, 69
ALA, food sources of, 55
Alcohol, 36, 87, 91–94
Al Fresco chicken sausages, 41
Almonds
  Almond-Crusted Chicken, 102
Alternating sets, in weight workouts, 150
Alvarado Street Bakery, 66
Alzheimer's disease, fish preventing, 40
American paradox, saturated fat and, 231
Anger management, fish oil for, 55
Angiotensinogen, high blood pressure
      from, 215
Antioxidants
  in avocados, 45
  in beverages for hydration, 87
  in coffee, 88
  phytochemicals as, 44
  for preventing vision problems, 41
  in tea, 89
Appetizers, in restaurant meals, 50
Arm circles, in dynamic warmup, 154, **154**
Arterial inflammation, from interleukin-6,
      215

Arthritis, fish oil preventing, 55
Artichokes
  Sautéed Baby Artichokes, 124
Artificial sweeteners, 90
Asiago cheese
  Chicken with Pancetta and Asiago, 106
Asparagus
  Tuscan Rib-Eye Steak and Prosciutto-
      Wrapped Asparagus, 127
Asthma, fish and fish oil preventing, 40, 55
At Large Nutrition Nitrean, 80
At Large Nutrition Opticen, 81
Avocados
  Avocado and Tomato Salad, 120
  as natural fat, 45

B

Back extension, in weight workout, 164,
      164
Bacon, 41
Bagels, recommended brand of, 67
Baked beans, 68
Balance, in total-body training, 141–44
Barbecue sauce, 49, 69
Barbell bent-over row, in weight workout,
      165, **165**
Barbell squat, in weight workout, 166,
      166
Barilla Plus pasta, 67
Beans, recommended types of, 68
Bear Naked All Natural Low Sugar
      Cereal, 69
Beef. *See also* Steak
  Asian Steak Stew, 117
  Beef Kebabs, 118
  Burritos, 128
  Chili, 121
  Cilantro Flank Steak, 119
  Filet Mignon with Tomato and
      Mozzarella Salad, 122
  health benefits from, 39
  as high-quality protein, 39, 59

V

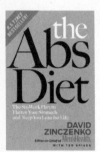

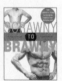

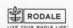